Words of Praise for
Reach for the Top

A pioneer in the exploding field of bioinformatics, mathematician/ physician Dr. W. John Wilbur, in a collection of erudite essays, presents the scientific evidence and describes his highly personal journey in quest of a better life.

He considers a variety of factors that will contribute to better health and a higher quality of life, including a simpler, more nutritious diet, exercise, rest, and abstinence from harmful habits. Much of this useful advice, in fact, was recommended long ago (at a time when medicine was influenced by science of varied veracity) by the writings of Ellen G. White, a founder of the Seventh-day Adventist Church, and continues to inspire the health mission of that organization.

~ **Philip S. Chen,** Jr, Ph.D., *Associate Director for Intramural Affairs, National Institutes for Health (retired)*

෯ ෬

When I seek medical advice, I try to find a doctor who keeps up on research. Though opinions are at times worthwhile, I want to know what research contributes. Dr. Wilbur does an excellent job of using research to add a wealth of information to the health topics about which he writes. The subjects are interesting and practical. I highly recommend his book.

~ **George Gibson,** PhD., *Emeritus Professor of American History and Economics at Union College*

෯ ෬

I have thoroughly enjoyed reading the information in this book. The author brings together years of research behind modern medicine and the tried and true health message of the Seventh-day Adventists. As a still learning and always seeking great grandmother it was a blessing to find trustworthy answers to my many health and spiritual questions.

~ **Katherine L. Schyllander**

ಇ ಚಿ

Solid. Factual. Well researched. Authentic. Personal. And, spiritual. If these words and phrases are attractive to you then you will enjoy this book. Dr. Wilbur, or as I know him, John, is a man of highest integrity and possesses a wealth of health knowledge. Never overbearing or judgmental, John simply shares the facts regarding health, nutrition and their relation to spiritual things. And he shares his own journey, even though some of its details may surprise. Trade drama for simple facts. Read this book!

~ **Pastor Dave VandeVere,** *VP-Finance at Mid-America Union of Seventh-day Adventists*

ಇ ಚಿ

Reach for the Top

Applying Adventist Health Principles in the Modern World

℅ ❖ ℬ

W. John Wilbur, MD, PhD

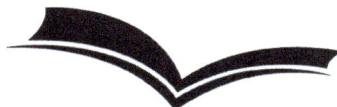

TEACH Services, Inc.
P U B L I S H I N G
www.TEACHServices.com • (800) 367-1844

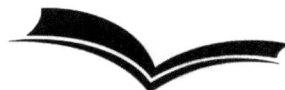

Copyright © 2024 W. John Wilbur, MD, PhD
Copyright © 2024 TEACH Services, Inc.
Published in Calhoun, Georgia, USA
ISBN-13: 978-1-4796-1776-0 (Paperback)
ISBN-13: 978-1-4796-1777-0 (ePub)
Library of Congress Control Number: 2024923409

Published by:

TEACH Services, Inc.
P U B L I S H I N G
www.TEACHServices.com • (800) 367-1844

Dedication

This book is dedicated to my dear wife, Bonnie, who encouraged me and also brought her expertise to bear in reading, editing, and making suggestions for improvements. The book is better for her efforts.

Table of Contents

Acknowledgement

I am grateful to Phil Chen, George Gibson, Mical Keaton, John Raymond, Kathy Schyllander, and Dave VandeVere for reading the book, and to Kathy Pflugrad at TEACH Services, Inc., for expertly guiding the book through the editing process.

Introduction

Seventh-day Adventists have become known in the medical science community through at least five Adventist health studies (Berkel & de Waard 1983; Fonnebo 1992; Fraser & Shavlik 2001; Oliveira et al. 2016; Orlich et al. 2013). All these studies have demonstrated the benefit of following the health teachings of the church. Of these studies, the two involving USA individuals have the advantages of larger sample sizes and including more information on risky or health-protective behaviors of the individuals in the study.

The first Adventist health study was of 34,192 non-Hispanic White Californians who were at least 30 years of age. They were followed from 1976–1988. Based on this study, it was concluded that those adherent to "high physical activity, frequent consumption of nuts, vegetarian status, and medium body mass index" and without a history of smoking enjoyed approximately a ten-year increase in life expectancy when compared with their peers (Fraser & Shavlik 2001).

A second domestic Adventist health study recruited participants between 2002 and 2007, resulting in 73,308 individuals throughout the USA. The focus was dietary patterns, mainly vegetarian versus nonvegetarian. Results showed a clear advantage, with Adventist vegetarians being 12% less likely to die during the study period than nonvegetarian Adventists were (Orlich et al. 2013).

What is interesting is the Adventist emphasis on health originated largely with a young woman by the name of Ellen G. White (1827–1915), who had no training in health science but claimed to have a message on the subject from God. Her writings on the subject began around 1864 and ended around 1909. Whatever one may think of White's beliefs and teachings on religious topics, her writings on health do have this testimony: little that was written about health in her day has endured, but her counsels on health have been found to be of enduring value.

Professor Clive M. McCay (1898–1967), of Cornell University, was introduced to the writings of Ellen White on health by one of his students in a History of Nutrition course. Dr. McCay's expertise was biochemistry, nutrition, and gerontology. He pioneered the first studies on calorie reduction and longevity (McDonald & Ramsey 2010). After studying her writings, he was puzzled. While he was suspicious of her claim to have a message from God, he could not explain her ability to produce what she wrote.

Dr. McCay summed up his reaction in four points: First, where did she obtain such enlightenment? He rejected the suggestion that she simply borrowed her ideas from others. He reacted, 'But how would she know which ideas to borrow and which to reject out of the bewildering array of theories and health teachings current in the nineteenth century? She would have had to be a most amazing person, with knowledge beyond her times, in order to do this successfully!' Second, how was she able to convince a substantial number of people to improve their diets? Third, he believed many more could have benefited in her day had they practiced what she taught. Finally, he questioned, 'How could her teachings be more widely disseminated to benefit future generations?' (Nichol 1964).

> *Much is known about life habits and how they impact health; we can all improve. It is our hope that you find benefit from reading these pages.*

Because you are reading these words, it is assumed you are interested in improving your health. It is the purpose of the author to assist you in reaching that goal. Herein, we present basic health principles as supported by scientific evidence and compare these with the teachings of Ellen White. This is in keeping with her instruction: "Our workers should use their knowledge of the laws of life and health. They should study from cause to effect. Read the best authors on these subjects, and obey religiously that which your reason tells you is truth" (1923). Much is known about life habits and how they impact health; we can all improve. It is our hope that you find benefit from reading these pages.

CHAPTER 1

Measuring Health

A time-honored definition of "health" is simply "absence of disease or injury." The World Health Organization has put forward a more inclusive definition: "Health is a state of complete physical, mental and social well-being and not merely the absence of disease or infirmity." While these are interesting and provocative definitions, they both have a fundamental lack. They are imprecise and difficult to apply in practice. In many cases, we could be confronted with two sick people and have no way to say whether one is healthier than the other is.

Medical science has defined a huge number of signs (what the doctor sees), symptoms (of which the patient complains), laboratory values, and radiological findings to characterize abnormalities in the human system, but no way to integrate these into a linear scale representing the level of health. To study a disease and discover methods of treating it, scientists must agree on when that disease is present. This has led to many diseases being defined by ad hoc collections of signs, symptoms, laboratory values, and radiological findings.

For example, "metabolic syndrome" is defined as having any three of the following five conditions: a large waistline, a high triglyceride level, a low HDL cholesterol level, high blood pressure, and high blood sugar. In practice, these conditions are more precisely defined (NHLBI, https://1ref. us/byb01, [accessed April 18, 2024]). Similarly, "major depression" is defined as the presence of at least five symptoms out of a longer list (NIMH, https://1ref.us/byb02, [accessed April 18, 2024]).

While such an approach to the characterization of a disease or syndrome provides a definition on which stakeholders can agree, it has a downside. It generally leaves a grey area where patients come close but do not quite satisfy the definition. Then one cannot say whether treatments found useful for those satisfying the definition are appropriate for those in the grey area. This is important because most treatments produce side effects (abnormalities) that must be weighed against the benefits of the treatment. In many cases, the treatment is to be desired, but in notable cases (e.g., fenfluramine-phentermine combination, rosiglitazone), the long-term effects of a treatment have proved damaging. We don't bring these issues up to disparage medical science, but rather to highlight the complexities and difficulties of the common approach. Any approach that hopes to improve the health of humanity will necessarily require some way of measuring health. As philanthropist Bill Gates said, "I have been struck again and again by how important measurement is to improving the human condition."

There is another and (we think) improved way to look at health. By analogy, consider a race car. To understand how well it works we might subject the different parts of the car, especially the engine, to many tests to see whether they were correctly constructed using the correct measurements. We could apply tests to see if the fuel injection system is working properly, and likewise for the spark plugs, oil pump, coolant pump, etc. We could check tire pressure, bearing lubrication, and timing belt. On the other hand, we could simply ask, What is the top speed of the car? That single test would give us a great deal of information in an uncomplicated way.

We could call this "performance testing." It even has the advantage of providing a linear scale along which the health of the car is measured. If the car does poorly on the performance test, then it may be necessary to get into detailed testing of the various parts of the engine and other subsystems. However, for many purposes, performance is what matters; if it is good, one need go no further. In the same way, we can think of performance testing the human body. There are a couple of ways such testing is applied in the field of medicine. One of these is by measuring longevity. Many treatments are evaluated by their effect on mortality. Clearly, longevity is the goal, and life span the measure of it. While measuring longevity has very important uses, it also has serious limitations. It is of no help in measuring the health of the individual patient as we only know the value when the patient has expired.

In some ways, a more useful performance measure for humans is peak exercise capacity (cardiorespiratory fitness or aerobic fitness). This is the peak rate at which an individual can burn oxygen metabolically. It has been found that the higher the peak exercise capacity, the lower the person's risk of dying. This relationship persists even to the very high fitness levels of elite athletes and remains true in old age (Mandsager et al. 2018). Since it makes sense that one could only achieve a high aerobic fitness if all the systems of the body were working well and well together, it makes sense that aerobic fitness is a good measure of health. The fact that aerobic fitness has a strong inverse relation with the risk of dying provides good supporting evidence.

While aerobic fitness has desirable features as a measure of health, it is not always available. It is difficult to measure in the elderly and frail or those who are ill. Another measure that has been examined is grip strength. This has the advantage of being easy to measure, even for the aged and many of those with suboptimal health. Grip strength has been found to be a good surrogate for muscular strength in general and strongly and inversely related to all causes of mortality as well as a large number of adverse health outcomes (Celis-Morales et al. 2018). Specifically, it is strength and not muscle mass that is measured and has the best inverse correlation with negative health outcomes (Newman et al 2006). Again, strength is a believable performance measure in that it depends on the health of the nerves and muscles and all the systems on which they are dependent as well.

It is interesting to compare our discussion with statements made by Ellen White regarding health. "Right physical habits promote mental superiority. Intellectual power, physical strength, and longevity depend upon immutable laws. There is no happen-so, no chance, about this matter. Nature's God will not interfere to preserve men from the consequences of violating nature's laws" (1954, p. 396). White was a spiritual leader and helped found the Seventh-day Adventist Church. She often spoke of spiritual concerns in her statements regarding physical health; she saw physical health as important to spiritual success.

The nineteenth century was a time when many believed in the theory known as "vitalism," i.e., "a doctrine that the functions of a living organism are due to a vital principle distinct from physicochemical forces" (*Merriam-Webster's Dictionary*, s.v. "vitalism"). As far as we have seen, White never used the term "vitalism." She did use the term "vital force," which is sometimes equated with vitalism, but she used it with the meaning of "force that prolongs life," as is it is commonly understood today. Note the following statement:

> God endowed man with so great vital force that he has withstood the accumulation of disease, brought upon the race in consequence of perverted habits, and he has continued for six thousand years. This fact of itself is enough to evidence to us the strength and electrical energy God gave to man at his creation. It took more than two thousand years of crime and indulgence of base passions to bring bodily disease upon the race to any great extent. If Adam, at his

creation, had not been endowed with twenty times as much vital force as men now have, the race, with present habits of living in violation of natural law, would have become extinct. ("Degeneracy— Education," *The Health Reformer*, November 1, 1872)

Historical records show that the average life span in the USA in 1870 was about 40 years. Multiply 40 by 20, and we obtain 800. Since Adam lived to 930 years, according to Genesis 5:5, if we measure vital force by length of life, we see the statement that Adam was endowed with twenty times the vital force of humanity in White's day is justified. She further held that by poor life habits, one could waste one's vital force:

> Everyone who violates the laws of health must sometime be a sufferer to a greater or less degree. God has provided us with constitutional force, which will be needed at different periods of our life. If we recklessly exhaust this force by continual overtaxation, we shall sometime be losers. Our usefulness will be lessened, if not our life itself destroyed. (*Counsels on Health*, p. 99)

> None can live when their vital energies are used up. They must die. (*A Solemn Appeal*, p. 74)

In summary, we see that Ellen White taught that strength and longevity were correlated measures of health in harmony with modern medical science. However, she added intellectual power as another measure of health correlated with strength and longevity. She further taught that all three of these elements would be prematurely diminished by reckless life habits.

White was not only concerned about health, strength, and longevity, but also how these factors affected one's usefulness and productivity. She gave an estimate of the damaging effects of intemperate eating by gospel ministers who partook of unhealthful dishes at the urging of parishioners. "They err when they tempt the minister with unhealthful food. Precious talent has thus been lost to the cause of God; and many, while they do live, are deprived of half the vigor and strength of their faculties" (1938, p. 55).

Speaking more broadly, White stated, "Through intemperance some sacrifice one half, and others two thirds of their physical, mental, and moral powers and become playthings for the enemy" (1954, p. 394). In her younger years, White endured poor health, but when she had received the message of health reform, she began to practice its principles. She witnessed a dramatic improvement in her health and strength:

I have fainted away with my child in my arms again and again. I have none of this now; and shall I call this a privation, when I can stand before you as I do this day? There is not one woman in a hundred that could endure the amount of labor that I do. I moved out from principle, not from impulse. I moved because I believed Heaven would approve of the course I was taking to bring myself into the very best condition of health, that I might glorify God in my body and spirit, which are His. (*Counsels on Diets and Foods*, p. 484)

In witness of her work ethic, Ellen White left over 25 million handwritten words and 100,000 printed and handwritten pages upon her death at age 87 (Coon 1998, p. 23). At the age of 81, she was still very active:

I am now in my eighty-first year, and I can bear testimony that we do not, as a family, hunger for the fleshpots of Egypt. I have known something of the benefits to be received by living up to the principles of health reform. I consider it a privilege as well as a duty to be a health reformer....

I consider that one reason why I have been able to do so much work both in speaking and in writing, is because I am strictly temperate in my eating. (*Counsels on Diets and Foods*, pp. 492, 493).

> *White left over 25 million handwritten words and 100,000 printed and handwritten pages upon her death at age 87.*

The best summary of healthy life habits in the medical literature of which I am aware is contained in the *Lifestyle Medicine Handbook*, produced in collaboration with the American College of Lifestyle Medicine. It presents "exercise, nutrition, sleep, smoking cessation, social connection, and mind-body health" as the six pillars of lifestyle medicine (Frates et al. 2019, p. 23).

Pure air, sunlight, abstemiousness, rest, exercise, proper diet, the use of water, trust in divine power—these are the true remedies. Every person should have a knowledge of nature's remedial agencies and how to apply them. It is essential both to understand the principles involved in the treatment of the sick and to have a practical training that will enable one rightly to use this knowledge. (White, *The Ministry of Healing*, p. 127)

Since White counseled strongly against the use of alcohol, tobacco, and drugs of abuse prevalent in her day (1949), we see much in common with the modern view. The goal is optimal health, and the challenge is to incorporate the laws of health in our daily practice. While we cannot claim to be perfect in our understanding or practice, she had some sage advice for anyone making the attempt:

> Why will not men and women to whom God has given reasoning powers exercise their reason? When they see their strength is failing, why do they not investigate their habits and their diet, and change to a different diet to see its effect? The sufferings that have been brought about by a so-called health reform have militated greatly against true reforms. These narrow ideas and this overstraining in the diet question have done great injury to physical, mental, and moral strength. (*The Retirement Years,* p. 128)

We believe this is excellent advice, not only regarding dietary matters, but also helpful in evaluating any change in life habits. Especially for one who partakes in regular exercise, it is not difficult to rate the effect of a change on one's energy level.

CHAPTER 2

A Simple Diet

To better understand the meaning and importance of a simple diet, we first need to understand something of the health challenges our world faces. The world is currently amid an obesity pandemic that continues to worsen, especially in middle- and low-income populations. The worldwide adult obesity rate nearly tripled between 1975 and 2016. During the same period, the childhood and adolescent (ages 5–19) obesity rate increased by a factor greater than six (Bluher 2019; N. C. D. Risk Factor Collaboration 2017). In 2016. the world's adult obesity rate was 13%, with an additional 27% classed as overweight. We can be sure both rates are higher now (World Health Organization, https://1ref.us/byb03, June 9, 2021).

High-income countries already have very high rates of obesity. The USA leads the way with a current adult obesity rate of 42.4% (Centers for Disease Control and Prevention, https://1ref.us/byb04, [last reviewed May 17, 2022]). Obesity is a risk factor for many non-infectious diseases and has been estimated to decrease life expectancy between 5 and 20 years depending on coexisting health problems (Bluher 2019). Obesity is defined in terms of BMI (Body Mass Index—height-adjusted version of a person's weight; it is defined as a person's weight in kilograms divided by height in meters squared.) An adult is classed as obese if one's BMI is above 30.

What is driving such a remarkable change in the world's population? Some might wish to point fingers at our genes, but the change is much too rapid to be a consequence of genetic changes. Furthermore, an extensive analysis of UK Biobank data has only been able to assign about 5% of variation in the population's BMI values to a genetic cause (Sulc et al. 2020), and that, even if it is changing, cannot change on a time scale relevant to the obesity pandemic. The same study did find evidence that 1.9% of the variation in BMI values appears to be due to the interaction of genetics and environment, but this is too small to provide significant help.

Researchers at Stanford University looked at a large number of people—some of whom had genetic variations thought most likely to predispose to weight gain—and found that these people were just as likely to be successful at losing weight as were people without these genetic variations (Gardner et al. 2018). This also suggests that genes have little to do with weight gain or loss for most people. Evidently, we must consider a changing environment as the basis for the world's weight problem.

Clearly, there is an imbalance between energy intake and energy expenditure; the question is, Are we eating too much or exercising too little? While exercise has decreased beginning circa 1910 with the invention of mechanized transportation and many labor-saving devices, much of this development predates the obesity pandemic, which began circa 1970 in the USA (Bluher 2019; Swinburn et al. 2011). In the four decades from 1970–2010, there was a remarkable increase in calorie consumption for the average American adult of 200–400 additional kcal/day (Wright et al. 2004; Bentley 2017; DeSilver 2016). The evidence points strongly in the direction of too great an energy intake, not just in the USA, but globally (Bluher 2019; Swinburn et al. 2011).

How can we understand the increase in energy consumption? We turn to the groundbreaking research of Professor Barbara Rolls of Pennsylvania State University, who discovered that people eat about the same weight of food at a meal to be satisfied from one meal to the next (Rolls 2010; 2013). For almost any dish that one enjoys, there is a lower-calorie version that weighs the same and is just as satisfying yet less threatening to the waistline. This discovery led Professor Rolls to her famous "Volumetrics" diet based largely on the fact that fruits, vegetables, and soups have high water content, are relatively low in calories, and yet are satisfying. High water content is important as it adds weight to a product without adding calories.

Therefore, we need to learn to think of our food in terms of energy density. How many calories are there per gram of food? For commercial products, one just needs to look at the nutrition facts label. There, one is told how many grams equal a serving and how many calories a serving contains. Then a simple division of calories by grams provides the energy density. As Dr. Neal Barnard says, "If one serving has fewer calories than grams, it is a good choice" (2018). That would be less than one calorie per gram and indeed a great choice for weight control. The real problem with the world's energy consumption is that too many people eat too much food with a high calorie density.

The calorie density of food is extremely important and relates very much to the concept of a simple diet. Most fruits, vegetables, and legumes naturally have a lower calorie density: below one calorie per gram. Healthy 100% whole grain bread can have as low as two calories per gram. Most undried nuts and seeds have about six calories per gram. Pure sugar is four calories per gram; pure fat or oil is nine calories per gram. The food industry has discovered that if they process the food to remove much of the fiber, vitamins, and minerals and add generous amounts of fat, sugar, and salt, people will buy more of their products. Such products are not simple; the processes are often complicated and highly technical. Our ancestors did not prepare food in this manner, but today, the food industry is highly competitive; therefore, innovation to produce the most appetizing food for the lowest price seems a matter of survival.

As a way of responding to the food industry, a group of researchers at the University of Sao Paulo in Brazil have proposed the NOVA food classification system (Monteiro et al. 2018). Four categories are defined:

- **Group 1: Unprocessed or minimally processed foods.** Mostly natural products, only processed to the extent required for preservation.

- **Group 2: Processed culinary ingredients.** Simple things such as oils, butter, sugar, and salt, used to make appetizing dishes.

- **Group 3: Processed foods.** Combinations of Group 1 and Group 2 ingredients to make simple dishes as is common in home cooking.

- **Group 4: Ultra-processed foods.** Generally, "industrial formulations manufactured from substances derived from foods or synthesized from other organic sources. They typically contain little or no whole foods, are ready-to-consume or heat up, and are fatty, salty or sugary and depleted in dietary fibre, protein, various micronutrients and other bioactive compounds. Examples include: sweet, fatty or salty packaged snack products, ice cream, sugar-sweetened beverages, chocolates, confectionery, French fries, burgers and hot dogs, and poultry and fish nuggets" (Monteiro et al. 2018; *Food systems and diets: Facing the challenges of the 21st century*, p. 37).

The term "ultra-processed" has gained some traction, presumably because it describes well some things that are wrong with the world's food supply (Chen et al. 2020; Elizabeth et al. 2020). Most studies of ultra-processed food have been observational but have shown a range of adverse health consequences, including increased cardiovascular diseases, several cancers, and obesity. No study has shown a health benefit from ultra-processed food (Elizabeth et al. 2020).

A recent randomized controlled trial of the effect of ultra-processed food versus unprocessed food found that a given person consumed ~500 calories/day more on an ultra-processed diet as opposed to an unprocessed diet (Hall et al. 2019). For each of the twenty people in the study, which diet was given first was randomly decided. This study was carried out on the metabolic ward of the Clinical Center at the National Institutes of Health in Bethesda, Maryland. It was carefully done with each diet lasting fourteen days. The energy density of the non-beverage portion of the ultra-processed diet was about two calories per gram, while that of the unprocessed diet was about one calorie per gram. This seems consistent with what one would expect from a diet based on energy-dense foods. An estimate of US food energy consumption as of 2010 placed the fraction coming from ultra-processed foods at 57.5% (Martinez Steele 2018). As often, the US seems to be the leader in this category, but other countries are closing the gap.

While the processing of food in removing fiber and important micronutrients clearly has its downside, processing does not tell the whole story. A study of 120,877 US men and women consisting of three cohorts followed for 12–20 years has provided some useful insights (Mozaffarian 2011). All participants were free of chronic diseases at the beginning of their participation, and none were obese. Scientists evaluated participants at four-year intervals and analyzed dietary factors to see which were significant in explaining weight changes.

Overall weight was observed to increase by 3.35 pounds per participant on average. For a minority, weight decreased. Major factors identified in the analysis to explain weight gain were increased consumption of French fries (+3.35 lb.), potato chips (+1.69 lb.), sugar-sweetened beverages (+1.00 lb.), unprocessed red meats (+0.95 lb.), processed red meats (+0.93 lb.), and boiled, baked, or mashed potatoes (+0.57 lb.). Potatoes and unprocessed red meat involve no processing, and French fries and potato chips involve little, so processing does not seem to be the issue, but rather the high calorie density.

We suspect the boiled, baked, or mashed potato category receives a bad rap here because of the sour cream or butter commonly included. On the flip side, major factors to explain weight loss were increased consumption of vegetables (-0.22 lb.), whole grains (-0.37 lb.), fruits (-0.49 lb.), nuts (-0.57 lb.), and yogurt (-0.82 lb.). Fruits, vegetables, and yogurt are easy to explain based on their low energy density. Whole grains eaten as hot or cold breakfast cereal generally have liquid added that provides low energy density. For example, rolled oats cooked in water and seasoned with milk and fruit can have an energy density below one calorie per gram. Whole grain bread will generally have an energy density of two or a little above, but the rich fiber content contributes to satisfying hunger and limiting how much one is likely to eat (Lattimer and Haub 2010). Perhaps it is surprising that nuts would contribute to weight loss. On the other hand, nuts are rich in fiber. Research suggests that the fiber reduces how much of the fat in nuts is digested (Hall et all 2019; Baer et al. 1997) and also satisfies hunger.

The biblical prescription for humanity's original diet is given in Genesis: "And God said, 'See, I have given you every herb *that* yields seed which *is* on the face of all the earth, and every tree whose fruit yields seed; to you it shall be for food'" (1:29). The text indicates mankind was to eat the fruits and seeds of plants. After sin entered, herbs of the field were added to their diet (see 3:18)—altogether a simple, natural diet that did not involve processing products to produce complicated mixtures of the things that grew.

"Grains, fruits, nuts, and vegetables constitute the diet chosen for us by our Creator. These foods, prepared in as simple and natural a manner as possible, are the most healthful and nourishing. They impart a strength, a power of endurance, and a vigor of intellect, that are not afforded by a more complex and stimulating diet" (White 1938, p. 81).

In Ellen White's day, food processing was not as sophisticated as it is today. Nevertheless, even in her day, she spoke against the effort put into creating dishes made from complicated mixtures of foods, especially those that involve a rich combination of foods and spices that would require a lot of time and, in the end, only be hurtful to one's health.

> All mixed and complicated foods are injurious to the health of human beings. Dumb animals would never eat such a mixture as is often placed in the human stomach....
>
> The richness of food and complicated mixtures of food are health destroying....
>
> Let them teach the people to preserve the health and increase the strength by avoiding the large amount of cooking that has filled the world with chronic invalids. By precept and example make it plain that the food which God gave Adam in his sinless state is the best for man's use as he seeks to regain that sinless state. (*Counsels on Diets and Foods*, pp. 113, 460).

How should we interpret these statements? Fortunately, we have some guidance:

> Let those who advocate health reform strive earnestly to make it all that they claim it is. Let them discard everything detrimental to health. Use simple, wholesome food. Fruit is excellent, and saves much cooking. Discard rich pastries, cakes, desserts, and the other dishes prepared to tempt the appetite. Eat fewer kinds of food at one meal, and eat with thanksgiving. (*Counsels on Diets and Foods*, p. 333)

Too much added oil or sugar makes food difficult to digest. The wrong combination of ingredients or a heavy use of spices may make a dish hard to assimilate. Some foods work well for one person and cause problems for another. Because of these differences, we are encouraged to learn what is best from experience:

> *Ultra-processed food and rich dishes that are difficult to digest deserve our concern.*

We must care for the digestive organs, and not force upon them a great variety of food. He who gorges himself with many kinds of food at a meal is doing himself injury. It is more important that we eat that which will agree with us than that we taste of every dish that may be placed before us. There is no door in our stomach by which we can look in and see what is going on; so we must use our mind, and reason from cause to effect. (*Counsels on Diets and Foods*, p. 111)

Evidence for the detrimental health effects of ultra-processed food is mounting. However, rich, complicated dishes that are difficult to digest also deserve our concern. As Solomon stated, "When you sit down to eat with a ruler, consider carefully what *is* before you; and put a knife to your throat if you *are* a man given to appetite. Do not desire his delicacies, for they *are* deceptive food" (Prov. 23:1–3). In Solomon's day the wealthy and powerful were the ones who could afford rich, complicated dishes designed to tempt the appetite, but those who partook would find they were deceived as they suffered the adverse health consequences. We can all benefit by limiting our food to more natural, simple options and, even on special occasions, being careful to limit dessert.

CHAPTER 3

Feeding Your Sweet Tooth

Most of us are very fond of dessert, which usually means something sweet. In fact, it does not have to be dessert. If it is sweet, we will likely find it tempting. Food manufacturers have caught on! It is estimated that 75% of the packaged foods available in food markets in the USA have sugar added (DiNicolantonio et al. 2016). It is thought that in 1750, the average Briton ate about four pounds of sugar per year; by 1850, twenty-five pounds per year (DiNicolantonio et al. 2016). The evidence suggests that today in the USA, the average adult eats about seventy-five pounds of added sugar per year (Bentley 2017). This might be well and good, but the evidence is it is killing a lot of us.

Data collected in the USA show that most Americans consume over 10% of their calories from added sugar (the average is around 15%). Compared with those who consume less than 10% of calories from added sugar, those who consume between 10% and 25% of calories as added sugar are 30% more likely to die, and those consuming over 25% are 2.75 times more likely to die (Yang et al. 2014). The evidence is strong that added sugar contributes to deaths from cardiovascular disease (DiNicolantonio et al. 2016; Yang et al. 2014; Temple 2018) and cancer (Hur et al. 2021; Makarem 2018).

We all know that fruits like apples, oranges, bananas, dates, figs, and strawberries are sweet and delicious when ripe. They do not represent added sugar and are healthy to eat. They contain sugar, but it is packaged with fiber and pectin to slow down digestion and absorption of the sugar and antioxidants to prevent oxidative damage. Added sugar is "naked" sugar without these protective substances. Added sugar causes damage in two broad ways: First, sugar, mostly in the form of sugar-sweetened beverages, does not satisfy the appetite, leading to weight gain (Malik and Hu 2022). Second, added sugars tend to be rapidly absorbed, elevating blood sugar levels and giving rise to increased oxidative stress (Colak et al. 2013; Esposito et al. 2002).

Evidence shows that had these sugars been accompanied by the natural protective fiber and antioxidants in whole fruits and vegetables, the oxidative stress would have been significantly reduced (Bacchetti et al. 2019; Chung et al. 2022; Cocate et al. 2014). Further steps on the pathway to disease are the development of systemic inflammation, insulin resistance, elevated blood lipids, and high blood pressure. These often culminate in heart disease, type 2 diabetes mellitus, or cancer (Malik and Hu 2022).

How excess weight, oxidative stress, and perhaps factors yet to be discovered contribute to the development of a diseased state is not yet fully understood. However, oxidized low-density lipoprotein (oxLDL) particles seem to play a key role in the development of coronary heart disease. LDL is familiar as the bad cholesterol; when oxidized, it is a potent cause of vascular damage (Jenkins et al. 2004). Among those with elevated oxLDL in their blood, 76% have coronary artery disease; conversely, 90% of those with coronary artery disease have an elevated level of oxLDL in their blood (DiNicolantonio et al. 2016). We conclude that oxidative stress plays a major role in the development of coronary heart disease.

Because sugar-sweetened beverages are a large part of the sugar problem in the USA (Yang et al. 2014), diet drinks with low-calorie artificial sweeteners have become quite popular to reduce added sugar intake. Whether diet drinks are a solution is a topic of considerable discussion (Malik and Hu 2022; Normand et al. 2021; Swithers 2016). Randomized trials seem to suggest if they are truly used as substitutes, they can lead to reduced sugar intake and weight loss. However, observational studies that simply look at how people use them suggest they are used more as add-ons with little if any benefit and possibly harm (Swithers 2016).

Fruit juice would seem to be safer than sugar-sweetened drinks are, but it is missing much of the natural fiber and nutrients; studies suggest it is also a health risk (Malik and Hu 2022). We all need to appreciate water for what it is: a very safe way to slake one's thirst. Data from the first Adventist Health Study showed that those who drank two or fewer glasses of water per day had roughly double the risk of a fatal coronary event compared to those who drank five or more glasses of water per day (Chan et al. 2002). Likely, those drinking little water were partaking of sugar-sweetened beverages.

Regarding what is healthy to drink, we have the witness of the prophet Daniel in his request: "Please test your servants for ten days, and let them give us vegetables to eat and water to drink" (1:12). We know the outcome of this diet: It produced robust health in the four Hebrew youth and a performance, said by King Nebuchadnezzar himself, to be ten times better than that of all the other trainees in the officer's training school (see verses 12–20).

Ellen White gave counsel on drinking: "In health and in sickness, pure water is one of Heaven's choicest blessings. Its proper use promotes health. It is the beverage which God provided to quench the thirst of animals and man. Drunk freely, it helps to supply the necessities of the system, and assists nature to resist disease.… Water is the best liquid possible to cleanse the tissues" (1938, pp. 419, 420). Note that "cleansing the tissues" is an internal thing.

Since God promised to bring His people "to a land flowing with milk and honey" (Exod. 3:8), it is clear He intends for His people to enjoy some sweetness. However, we also have this counsel: "*It is* not good to eat much honey" (Prov. 25:27).

Ellen White also advised carefully limiting added sugar in one's diet:

> Far too much sugar is ordinarily used in food. Cakes, sweet puddings, pastries, jellies, jams, are active causes of indigestion. Especially harmful are the custards and puddings in which milk, eggs, and sugar are the chief ingredients. The free use of milk and sugar taken together should be avoided.…
>
> I frequently sit down to the tables of the brethren and sisters, and see that they use a great amount of milk and sugar. These clog the system, irritate the digestive organs, and affect the brain. Anything that hinders the active motion of the living machinery, affects the brain very directly. And from the light given me, sugar, when largely used, is more injurious than meat. (*Counsels on Diets and Foods*, pp. 327, 328)

White made this last statement in 1870, long before scientific studies had established the danger of using too much sugar. Furthermore, the average use of sugar at that time was probably about a third of what it is today. The statement that sugar "largely used, is more injurious than meat" seems to accord with the observation that sugar is a greater cause of cardiovascular disease than saturated fat is (DiNicolantonio et al. 2016; Temple 2018).

White's statements above regarding sugar contain a warning that sugar causes indigestion. This is not an issue that seems to interest the research community. After all, there seem to be far greater problems that threaten health. Why should we believe that foods rich in sugar cause indigestion?

What we do know is a water-based solution can only move from the stomach to the small bowel at a rate limited by the number of particles other than water in the solution. This limits the movement of the common sugar sucrose from the stomach to the duodenum to about a gram per minute (Kim et al. 2013).

We do not know if this is important in explaining the problem with sugar, but it does seem to be important. With certain types of stomach surgery, the mechanism that limits the flow of particles in solution to the small bowel is no longer functional. In that case, both solid meals and solutions with sugar in them can move freely and quickly from the stomach to the small bowel. This does not pose a problem when it is solid food consisting of relatively large particles that do not generate much osmotic force.

However, when a concentrated solution with many sugar molecules or salt ions moves freely into the small intestine, the particles exert a strong osmotic force to move water from the bloodstream into the intestine. This can be very uncomfortable with sweating, palpitations, faintness, etc. due to a drop in blood pressure, followed by the body's hormonal response known as "dumping syndrome." Part of the treatment for dumping syndrome is changing what one eats. The following is a statement by the National Institute of Diabetes and Digestive and Kidney Diseases regarding dumping syndrome:

> Your doctor may recommend
> - eating more protein, fiber, and fat
> - eating less carbohydrates and choosing foods that contain complex carbohydrates—such as whole grains, fruits, and vegetables—rather than foods that contain simple sugars—such as candies, cookies, sugary drinks, and other foods and drinks that have added sugar
> - avoiding milk and milk products
> - adding pectin or guar gum—plant extracts used as thickening agents—to your food (https://1ref.us/byb16, [last reviewed January 2019])

Clearly, added sugar is singled out, as well as milk and milk products. The normal stomach would prevent these foods from moving too quickly into the small intestine, but after a partial gastrectomy, the valve at the bottom of the stomach often no longer works properly, and dumping syndrome results. Conversely, notice that whole grains, fruits, and vegetables do not cause a problem. The important conclusion here is the normal stomach can allow foods like whole grains, fruits, and vegetables to enter the small bowel rapidly, but it holds back the flow of free sugars and milk products. Ellen White is basically saying this holding back is giving these foods time to ferment and cause indigestion: "Sugar clogs the system. It hinders the working of the living machine" (1938, p. 327).

How then should we deal with added sugar? Ellen White counsels that we will be healthier and have clearer minds if we limit it to a small amount. She herself practiced this advice:

> *Fruit pie is preferred because much of the sugar is from the fruit and has the natural fiber, pectin, and antioxidants with it.*

- "We have always used a little milk and some sugar.…"

- "Plain, simple pie may serve as dessert…"

- "Eggs can be prepared in a variety of ways. Lemon pie should not be forbidden."

- "The dessert should be placed on the table and served with the rest of the food; for often, after the stomach has been given all it should have, the dessert is brought on, and is just that much too much" (1938, pp. 330–334).

We recommend fruit pie over cake, sweet bread, and other grain-based desserts. We have found that one can often reduce the added sugar from what is listed in a recipe. Fruit pie is preferred because much of the sugar is from the fruit and has the natural fiber, pectin, and antioxidants with it. On the other hand, cake or sweet bread is generally made from highly processed flour, which is missing the fiber and has all the sugar added. Even better than fruit pie is fresh fruit when available.

CHAPTER 4

Fats—Healthy and Unhealthy

Fats are important ingredients in some of the most delectable dishes one can imagine, but in the recent past, it was considered gospel truth that to be healthy, one needed to eat a low-fat diet. Happily, the evidence has freed us from that notion (Willett 2012). However, increasing the amount of fat by eating more animal products increases the likelihood of death from any cause as well as cardiovascular mortality, but increasing fat by eating more plants decreases those likelihoods and cardiovascular mortality (Seidelmann et al. 2018). Animal products are high in saturated fat while plants are high in unsaturated fat.

Despite much research, opinions vary as to what kind of unsaturated fat is best (DiNicolantonio and O'Keefe 2017; Ramsden et al. 2009; Sacks 2017). However, there is a strong consensus that trans fats should be completely avoided, and saturated fats should be strictly limited for the healthiest diet (Willett 2012; DiNicolantonio and O'Keefe 2017; Ramsden et al. 2009; Sacks 2017). For the last fifty years, this view has rested largely on the "cholesterol hypothesis," which posits that atherosclerosis is a consequence of elevated LDL cholesterol in the blood. This doctrine has recently been severely criticized (DuBroff 2017; DuBroff and de Lorgeril 2015; Ravnskov et al. 2020; Ranvskov et al. 2018), and the value of using drugs to lower cholesterol has been challenged. However, the evidence that lowering cholesterol reduces cardiovascular disease and death is strong and comes from multiple sources (Chen et al. 2022; Chowdhury et al. 2013; Esselstyn 2014; Ference et al. 2017; Goldstein and Brown 2015). We believe the more relevant questions are, When does cholesterol need to be lowered? and what is the healthiest way to accomplish this? As we will see, the contribution of fats to the cholesterol problem is incompletely understood.

Evidence of the harmful effects of industrially produced trans fats comes from short-term studies of human physiology, showing not only an increase in LDL cholesterol levels and a decrease in HDL cholesterol levels but also an increase in serum triglycerides as well as an indication of systemic inflammation seen in elevated levels of C-reactive protein, interleukin-6, and tumor necrosis factor alpha (Willett 2012; Mozaffarian et al. 2006). There is also evidence from a pooled analysis of observational studies that an increase of 2% in trans-fat calories is associated with a 29% increase in coronary heart disease (Mozaffarian et al. 2006). Evidence of the mechanism for damage from physiologic studies, coupled with evidence of damage in those with higher intake, makes for strong evidence of causality. This has led to the settled opinion that trans fats are damaging, so it would be unethical to conduct long-term human studies of the effect of trans fats on human health (Mozaffarian et al. 2006).

Saturated fats represent a more complicated problem. First, it is important to point out that intake of saturated fats at a low level has not been shown to be damaging. The common plant-derived cooking oils range from 6–17% saturated (Sacks et al. 2017). Almonds have 10% of the fat as saturated; cashews, 20%; filberts, 7%; walnuts, 11%; and peanuts, 14% (Pennington 1989). On the other hand, animal fats tend to be highly saturated: haddock, 32%; chicken, 35%; pork, 40%; mutton, 48%; beef, 50%; and butter, 63% (Sacks et al. 2017; Beare 1962).

At the time of this writing, the American Heart Association recommends limiting intake of saturated fat to less than 10% of calories eaten. This recommendation is based on the observation that saturated fat raises LDL cholesterol, and the assumption is the cholesterol hypothesis is true (Sacks et al. 2017). For most foods, saturated fatty acids are mainly palmitate and stearate. Stearate does not raise cholesterol; thus, the real culprit in elevating cholesterol is palmitate (Ramsden et al. 2009). However, both palmitate and stearate can cause lipotoxicity (Deguil et al. 2011; Lipke et al. 2022; Spigoni et al. 2017). Lipotoxicity occurs when cells are exposed to these fatty acids at elevated levels, and by means not well understood, such exposure triggers inflammation, disorders basic cell functions, and can ultimately cause cell death.

Lipotoxicity plays a fundamental role in type 2 diabetes (Eguchi et al. 2012), fatty liver disease (Ogawa et al. 2018), and cardiovascular diseases (Spigoni et al. 2017; Shen et al. 2013). Cells have built-in protection from lipotoxicity through the action of the enzyme stearoyl CoA desaturase, which converts palmitate and stearate to the unsaturated fatty acids palmitoleate and oleate (Oshima et al. 2020; Stamatikos et al. 2013). They also appear to be protected by simply having enough of the unsaturated fatty acids palmitoleate or oleate to counteract the presence of palmitate and stearate (Oshima et al. 2020; Nolan and Larter 2009; Leamy et al. 2016). The means by which the presence of these monounsaturated fatty acids protect against lipotoxicity is not yet understood.

The fact that there are protective mechanisms makes it understandable that low levels of saturated fat intake are not damaging. Damage comes when these protective mechanisms are overwhelmed. Normal, healthy people store fat in fat cells mostly located in a layer called "adipose tissue" between the skin and the muscles. When fat is needed as a fuel by other tissues, it is released in a controlled manner from the fat cells. If a person eats more calories than can be used by the body, the excess energy is stored as fat in the fat cells. As fat builds up, fat cells can swell in diameter up to 20 times with an increase in volume of several thousandfold. This can cause cells or even parts of cells to be too far from a blood vessel.

When this happens, cells can have insufficient oxygen to function normally (Halberg et al. 2009; Snel et al. 2012). In this state, cells begin to signal their distress, which attracts cells of the immune system, leading to inflammation. Some of these hypoxic cells will die. This results in further inflammation as the immune system is called in to clean up the remnants of dead cells. Fat overload can occur even when healthy fat is consumed. It only requires the system to be overloaded with too many calories. However, if saturated fat is consumed at a high level, the fat cells themselves suffer from similar effects, as seen in other cell types (lipotoxicity), and become overloaded with fat sooner. As they can no longer store the fat, it is dumped into the bloodstream and circulates to other tissues, where it begins to be retained (Lipke et al. 2022; Snel et al. 2012; Luukkonen et al. 2018; Kade et al. 2022; Takeda et al. 2021).

Feeding studies of humans given diets high in palmitate and stearate show a buildup of fat in the internal organs, especially the liver and pancreas but also the heart and muscles, resulting in elevated markers of inflammation and lipotoxicity (Luukkonen et al. 2018; Parry 2020; Rosqvist et al. 2014; Toledo et al. 2018). It is this buildup of fat in vital organs that is implicated in type 2 diabetes, fatty liver disease, and cardiovascular diseases (Lipke et al. 2022; Snel et al. 2012; Taylor 2008).

Having said that saturated fat is bad, it is reasonable to ask whether all forms of saturated fat are equally bad. Two studies have examined different sources of saturated fat to see if there is a difference in their health effects (de Oliveira et al. 2012; O'Sullivan et al. 2013). In both studies, the conclusion was reached that eating more dairy fat did not raise the risk, while eating more meat fat did raise the risk. One study focused on cardiovascular disease (CVD). Data from the Multi-Ethnic Study of Atherosclerosis

(MESA) were analyzed, with results showing a drop in risk of CVD by 25% if 2% of energy from meat fat was replaced with dairy fat (de Oliveira et al. 2012).

The other study was based on data from twenty-six prior studies (not including the MESA study). It concluded that those having the highest intake of dairy had no increased risk of death over those with the lowest dairy intake; whereas those with the highest intake of meat had a 17% increased risk of death, and those with the highest intake of processed meat had a 21% increased risk of death compared with those having the lowest intakes, respectively (O'Sullivan et al. 2013). Since both meat and dairy are high in saturated fat, this raises the question, What other substance or substances, either in dairy or meat, is making the difference? One possibility is that the L-carnitine in meat causes a change in the colonic bacteria, leading to the conversion of L-carnitine to trimethylamine, which is absorbed and converted in the liver to trimethylamine N-oxide (TMAO).

TMAO is a toxic substance that greatly increases the risk of atherosclerosis (Abbasi 2019). Not everyone produces TMAO from L-carnitine, but it has been found that meat eaters are ten times more likely to be high producers of TMAO compared to vegetarians (Wu et al. 2019). A second possibility is the intake of the heme iron in meat. An excess of iron in the liver contributes to insulin resistance and correlates with an increased risk of cardiovascular diseases (Haap et al. 2011; Hua et al. 2001; Zheng et al. 2011; de Oliveira et al. 2012). A third possibility is the medium-chain fatty acids in dairy (carbon backbones of length 6–12), which provide a measure of protection from lipotoxicity (Nagao and Yanagita 2010; Ronis et al. 2013; Schonfeld and Wojtczak 2016; Wang et al. 2017). Interestingly, these medium-chain fatty acids are found in significant amounts in animal milk but are almost completely absent from meat.

Certain unsaturated fatty acids, called "polyunsaturated" because they have more than one double bond in their carbon backbones, are essential to include in our diets because humans are unable to make them. One of these is named "linoleic acid" (omega-6) and is quite plentiful in plants. The other is named "alpha linolenic acid" (omega-3) and is less common in the plant world. In most plants and animal products, there is ten times as much linoleic acid as there is alpha linolenic acid. Exceptions where alpha linolenic acid is plentiful are flax seeds, chia seeds, English walnuts, and canola oil. From these essential fatty acids, our bodies make long-chain fatty acids that have important functions in human physiology. Alpha linolenic acid, which has 18 carbons in length, is used by our bodies to make eicosapentaenoic acid (EPA, 20 carbons) and docosahexaenoic acid

(DHA, 22 carbons). Docosahexaenoic acid is an important building block in the brain.

These two long-chain omega-3 fatty acids are also found in fatty fish such as salmon, herring, and sardines. It has become quite popular to take fish oil for its assumed health benefits. This has led to many studies testing whether fish oil might reduce heart disease, diabetes, depression, Alzheimer's disease, or cancer, among others. Unfortunately, there is very little convincing evidence that fish oil gives significant help with any of these major health problems (Abdelhamid et al. 2020; Brown et al. 2019; Burckhardt et al. 2016; Lee et al. 2020; Luo et al. 2020). Fish oil supplements represent a roughly $2 billion market globally, and it's only growing. This is money that might be better spent in most cases, though your doctor might prescribe fish oil to lower elevated triglycerides.

Another issue of importance is whether coconut oil is a health risk. Coconut contains almost completely saturated fat, but the fatty acids are mostly of medium chain length. Evidence is accumulating that these fatty acids can offer protection from lipotoxicity (Nagao and Yanagita 2010; Ronis et al. 2013; Schonfeld and Wojtczak 2016; Wang et al. 2017). Coconut oil has been shown to elevate LDL cholesterol, but that is of uncertain significance. Two island populations have been studied where coconuts comprise a major dietary energy source, yet these populations have almost no heart disease (Lindeberg et al. 1994; Stanhope and Prior 1976; Stanhope et al. 1981). Based on these facts, it is not clear that coconut oil increases cardiovascular risk (DiNicolantonio et al. 2017). Yet many remain convinced that coconut oil is not as healthy as unsaturated vegetable oils are (Abbasi 2020). It seems unlikely this issue will be completely settled without more study. In the meantime, moderation is always in order.

In the Old Testament Scriptures, Moses wrote of God's instruction to Israel:

> There He made a statute and an ordinance for them, and there He tested them, and said, "If you diligently heed the voice of the LORD your God and do what is right in His sight, give ear to His commandments and keep all His statutes, I will put none of the diseases on you which I have brought on the Egyptians. For I *am* the LORD who heals you." (Exodus 15:25, 26)

One thing we know about the Egyptians from the examination of mummies: they were afflicted with atherosclerosis (David et al. 2010), which is the fundamental pathology underlying most coronary heart disease and strokes. Examination of ancient documents suggests that the priestly class would have partaken largely of animal fat (*Ibid.*), and it was this class that could afford mummification. We do not know so much about the poorer classes in Egypt, but it does suggest there was no prohibition against eating animal fat.

By contrast, God said to the Israelites, "*This shall be* a perpetual statute throughout your generations in all your dwellings: you shall eat neither fat nor blood" (Lev. 3:17). "Speak to the children of Israel, saying: 'You shall not eat any fat. of ox or sheep or goat'" (7:23).

Ellen White goes even further in stating that God gave the Israelites all the instruction needed to be healthy both physically and spiritually. "God gave to Israel instruction in all the principles essential to physical as well as to moral health" (1905, p. 283). God not only instructed Israel not to partake of animal fat but gave them explicit instruction approving the eating of oil, which, at that time, would have been olive oil:

> And if you bring as an offering a grain offering baked in the oven, *it shall be* unleavened cakes of fine flour mixed with oil, or unleavened wafers anointed with oil. But if your offering *is* a grain offering *baked* in a pan, *it shall be of* fine flour, unleavened, mixed with oil. You shall break it in pieces and pour oil on it; it *is* a grain offering" (Leviticus 2:4–6).

Of such an offering, the priest would take a portion to burn on the altar, but the remainder was for the priest and his family to eat (see verses 7–10). Olive oil was an approved part of Israel's diet. We also observe that God promised Israel a land flowing with milk and honey, strongly implying that milk and cream were not forbidden foods (see Exod. 3:8).

White also gave instruction regarding the eating of fats. She recommended not eating any grease. Grease had the main meaning of "rendered animal fat" in her day. "You should keep grease out of your food. It defiles any preparation of food you may make" (1938, p. 354). She went further, decrying the increasing burden of disease in animals and the methods by which they are often prepared for market: "The liability to take disease is increased tenfold by meat eating" (p. 386).

However. White recommended milk and cream as part of a healthful diet: "Fruits, grains, and vegetables, prepared in a simple way, free from spice and grease of all kinds, make, with milk or cream, the most healthful diet" (p. 354). Nuts can also be part or a healthy diet. "Nuts and nut foods are coming largely into use to take the place of flesh meats. With nuts may be combined grains, fruits, and some roots, to make foods that are healthful and nourishing" (p. 363). With all this said, olives received her highest recommendation:

> Olives may be so prepared as to be eaten with good results at every meal....
>
> When properly prepared, olives, like nuts, supply the place of butter and flesh meats. The oil, as eaten in the olive, is far preferable to animal oil or fat. It serves as a laxative. Its use will be found beneficial to consumptives, and it is healing to an inflamed, irritated stomach. (*Counsels on Diet and Foods*, pp. 349, 350)

This statement on the benefits of olive oil finds some scientific support in a recent publication in the Nurses' Health Study and the Health Professionals Follow-Up Study (Guasch-Ferre et al. 2022). In these studies, a large number of US health professionals were followed for 28 years. It was found that those who consumed more than half a tablespoon (7 grams) of olive oil per day, when compared with those who rarely or never ate olive oil, were 19% less likely to die of cardiovascular disease, 17% less likely to die of cancer, 29% less likely to die of a neurodegenerative disease, and 18% less likely to die of a respiratory disease. The risk of dying was reduced by replacing margarine, butter, mayonnaise, and dairy fat with olive oil.

White also gave some cautions regarding fats, largely having to do with digestion:

> "Butter should not be placed on the table; for if it is, some will use it too freely, and it will obstruct digestion. But for yourself, you should occasionally use a little butter on cold bread, if this will make the food more appetizing. This would do you far less harm than to confine yourself to preparations of food that are not palatable....
>
> The grease cooked in the food renders it difficult of digestion....
>
> Three years ago a letter came to me saying, "I cannot eat the nut foods; my stomach cannot take care of them." Then there were several recipes presented before me; one was that there must be other ingredients combined with the nuts, which would harmonize with them, and not use such a large proportion of nuts. One-tenth to one-sixth part of nuts would be sufficient, varied according to combinations. We tried this, and with success. (*Counsels on Diet and Foods*, pp. 350, 354, 364)

We see two problems at issue here. First, we believe highly saturated fat, which is in solid form, is difficult to digest because digestion can only take place at the surface of this solid substance, which is relatively small. If the same fat were in an emulsion (e.g., cream), a much larger surface area is exposed to digestive enzymes, and the process can take place much faster (Drouin-Chartier et al. 2017; Guo et al. 2017; Peng et al. 2021). Second, even healthy fats are known to leave the stomach slowly, suggesting the digestive process is more time-consuming for fats than for other nutrients (Gentilcore et al. 2006; Kleibeuker et al. 1988). In medical school, I learned the rule of thumb that each additional ten grams of fat added to a meal delays the digestive process an additional hour. I believe this is a very useful rule. It warns us not to make our food too rich with fat or it will delay digestion to the point where the stomach will not be ready for the next meal.

Given the evidence, what should be recommended regarding the consumption of fats? The evidence seems clear that trans fats are harmful and should be avoided. Fortunately, they have virtually disappeared from store shelves since the 2013 ruling by the FDA that trans fats can no longer be designated "Generally Recognized as Safe" in human food. If there is a concern, check the ingredients list for the words "partially hydrogenated oil." If that is found, avoid the product, as it contains trans fat and is unsafe.

Why, if God gave the Israelites all the instruction needed to be healthy and the eating of meat is unhealthy, did not God prohibit the eating of meat?

We also recommend that meat be avoided when its place can be supplied by nuts, seeds, olives, and avocados. Both dairy and coconut oil are highly saturated, but both have an ample supply of short and medium-chain fatty acids that protect from lipotoxicity when used in moderation. For a cooking oil, we recommend olive oil above any other, as it has many health benefits, as already described. Assuming one eats a mostly plant-based diet, the need for linoleic acid and alpha linolenic acid will be naturally supplied—no need to take fish oil or extra omega-3 fatty acid supplements.

One may ask, Why, if God gave the Israelites all the instruction needed to be healthy and the eating of meat is unhealthy, did not God prohibit the eating of meat? Ellen White tells us, "Flesh was never the best food: but its use is now doubly objectionable, since disease in animals is so rapidly increasing" (1954, p. 382). This suggests that flesh was less of a health problem in ancient times but still not ideal. Though God did not command the Israelites to abstain from eating flesh, they did receive instruction indicating flesh was not the ideal food. Moses' writings gave the history of God's original dietary prescription for humanity, as well as the greatly shortened life span after the flood, when flesh was permitted as food.

Also, God's promise to the Israelites to heal them of their diseases (see Exod. 15:26) was made at the beginning of their wilderness wandering and followed shortly by the giving of the manna, which was to be their main sustenance. They experienced God's blessing in eating the manna and His hot displeasure when they demanded flesh to eat in place of the manna (see Numb. 11). God could not bless them with the spirit of rebellion in the camp, so He removed the ring leaders of the rebellion with a plague. After forty years on a diet mainly of manna, God, through Balaam, described them as blessed of God and having the strength of a wild ox (see 23:20, 22).

Interestingly, God provided quail as flesh for the complaining Israelites, which is believed to be not as damaging as red meat is, yet we are told, "And He gave them their request, but sent leanness into their soul" (Ps. 106:15). Apparently, quail and, by implication, chicken are not ideal as food.

What about eggs? Ellen White gave some counsel regarding eggs: "we should not consider it a violation of principle to use eggs from hens that are well cared for and suitably fed. Eggs contain properties that are remedial agencies in counteracting certain poisons" (1938, p. 352). While she does not specify the poisons mentioned here, the statement is clearly not referring to treating with eggs someone who has accidentally or intentionally imbibed a poison. The statement only makes sense if the poison is something that may be counteracted by using eggs on a regular basis. Considering this, we can point to lutein and zeaxanthin, which are powerful antioxidants prevalent in human nervous tissue, especially the retina.

Eggs are a rich source of these antioxidants. Those who eat eggs have been found to greatly reduce the risk of serious macular degeneration and blindness. The benefits may even extend to our cognitive abilities (Gopinath et al. 2020; Khalighi Sikaroudi et al. 2021; Stringham et al. 2019). One of the principal ways in which lutein and zeaxanthin are thought to benefit is by counteracting the toxic effects of oxygen free radicals (Stringham et al. 2019). It is true that egg consumption in the general population has been associated with some mortality risk (Zhong et al. 2019), but consuming up to four eggs per week was not associated with an increased risk of diabetes or mortality in Adventist Health Study 2 (Orlich et al. 2022; Sabate et al. 2018).

White made a point to recommend the use of milk and eggs only from healthy animals.

> While I would discard flesh meat as injurious, something less objectionable may be used, and this is found in eggs. Do not remove milk from the table or forbid its being used in the cooking of food. The milk used should be procured from healthy cows, and should be sterilized....
>
> I wish to say that when the time comes that it is no longer safe to use milk, cream, butter, and eggs, God will reveal this. No extremes in health reform are to be advocated. The question of using milk and butter and eggs will work out its own problem. At present we have no burden on this line. Let your moderation be known unto all men. (*Counsels on Diet and Foods*, p. 367)

Chapter 5

Satisfying Meals

Some people might think the most satisfying meal is the one where they eat all they want of everything they want. However, we have all learned by experience that does not lead to happiness but rather distress. Therefore, our goal here is to understand how we can have meals that are both healthy and satisfying. To this end, we believe there are basic principles that will reward us if they are followed. Expressed succinctly: eat food that is minimally processed; limit the times you eat; limit the variety at any one meal; and take time to eat and enjoy your food. It is the goal of this chapter to clarify and expand on these four basic principles.

Healthy food is minimally processed to preserve as much as possible of the natural fiber, vitamins, and minerals. If salt, sugar, or oil are added, they are added in limited quantities. It is recommended that men eat at least thirty-eight grams of fiber per day and women eat at least twenty-five, but the average intake in America is about half that. These levels are set with the goal to minimize the risk of heart disease, but fewer than 5% of Americans reach them (Jones 2014).

How does one know if a product has a healthy amount of fiber? Whole grain bread or cereal that is labeled 100% whole grain has all its fiber; barring other problems, it should be a healthy food. Many grain products are processed at some level; however, we can distinguish a healthy fiber level by examining the ingredients label. If the total carbohydrates in grams divided by ten is less than the total fiber in grams, that product has a healthy level of fiber (Mozaffarian et al. 2013). We find this to be a useful rule and recommend it. If a product must add back some of the vitamins or minerals that have been removed in processing, then it would be wise to look for a less processed version of that food.

"Salty" is one of the fundamental flavors. We all experience that a little salt adds significantly to the pleasure of eating. However, too much salt in our food increases blood pressure and cardiovascular risk. There is also much epidemiological evidence that high salt intake is associated with increased body weight (Zhang et al. 2016). Current guidelines for Americans recommend limiting sodium intake to fewer than 2,300 milligrams of sodium per day for those ages 14 and older (USDA/USDHHS 2020). Few Americans follow this guideline; the average American adult intake is around 3,500 milligrams of sodium per day (Sacks 2001).

It seems that people acquire a taste for salty food. Once the taste is acquired, less salty food is not very appealing. This is the result of purchasing ready-to-eat food with too much salt. The solution is to prepare one's own food or purchase food containing less salt. The goal is to prepare or purchase food that averages no more than 140 milligrams of sodium per serving (Cleveland Clinic, https://1ref.us/byb06, May 1, 2023). This is easily checked by examining nutrition labels on products purchased at the grocery store. Experiments show we can train ourselves through a reduction in salt intake to enjoy a diet with a reduced, healthier salt intake in as little as twelve weeks (Blais et al. 1986). My wife and I have put this into practice and find it works.

"Sweet" as a taste is a major source of pleasure and naturally results from the intake of various types of sugar. Sugar in the form of glucose or fructose is widely distributed in many kinds of fruit that can form a healthy part of one's diet. In this natural form, the sugar is packaged with fiber, pectin, antioxidants, and other substances that prevent damage. Risk to one's health surfaces when sugar without these protective substances is added to foods to make them more palatable. It seems to be unimportant whether the sugar is fructose, glucose, or common table sugar (disaccharide sucrose composed of equal parts fructose and glucose); the risk comes from overconsumption (Tappy and Le 2010).

The American Heart Association recommends limiting added sugars to 6% of calories consumed. We can relate this parameter to the one on healthy fiber mentioned above. If we divide the total carbohydrates by ten, we said the fiber in grams ought to be greater. Ideally, the added sugar in grams ought to be less or, at most, only a little more. This assumes one is eating a healthy diet with about 55% of calories from carbohydrates (Seidelmann et al. 2018) so that a tenth of the carbohydrates is about 6% of total calories. This is a useful rule of thumb to help steer you away from unhealthy products.

"Fat" is a taste; yes, we have taste buds that sense fatty acids in our food (Keast et al 2021). Such taste buds are located not only in the mouth but throughout the gastrointestinal tract. However, most of the fat we consume is in the form of triglycerides. One molecule of triglyceride is composed of three fatty acid molecules combined with a glycerol molecule. In this form, fat provides something called "mouthfeel," which is more a texture than it is a flavor (Keast et al 2021). During digestion, the triglycerides are broken down to fatty acids, and glycerol and the fatty acids are sensed by the fat-sensitive taste buds. Together, fat taste and mouthfeel make a large contribution to the palatability of food.

The problem with fat is it has nine calories per gram, while carbohydrates and proteins have only four calories per gram. The risk is we may be tempted to use too much fat in preparing our food. Food that is too calorie-dense is not healthy, even if the fat is healthy fat. Studies show that as a rule, the more calorie-dense our food is, the more we will weigh. Obese men and women eat food averaging 1.96 and 1.89 calories per gram, respectively, while lean men and women average 1.81 and 1.80 calories per gram, respectively (Vernarelli et al. 2015). Individuals will vary in what works for them, but these are reasonable guidelines.

Fresh fruit is generally well below one calorie per gram; even bananas and apricots packed in heavy syrup satisfy this rule. The same is true for fresh or frozen vegetables. We find that a little salt and some oil is sufficient to make vegetables palatable. The most calorie-dense vegetable I could find in our freezer is sweet corn, with seventy calories for an eighty-five-gram serving. For a twelve-ounce package, we add about two teaspoons of olive oil, and that brings the calorie density to 1.06 calories per gram. Cheerios with a cup of milk comes in at 0.63 calories per gram, and cooked cereal with milk and fruit is also lower than one calorie per gram. Bread is not much different from cooked cereal when properly chewed and should be counted no differently. If most of the food one eats is fruit, vegetables, and whole grains, then there is room for an entrée and even a dessert that are calorie-dense as long as the servings are reasonably sized.

Regarding entrees or desserts, we suggest that when possible, the fat be in the form of nut pieces. Studies show that almonds, even after chewing, are only partially digested. A significant amount of the fat is protected from digestion because the cells that contain it remain intact and the cell walls are resistant to digestive enzymes (Ellis et al 2004). This is true for roasted as well as raw almonds. Studies show that only about 80% of the fat in almonds and walnuts is digested and used by the body (McArthur and Mattes 2020). However, the same is presumably not true if the nuts are finely ground to make a nut butter (Capuano et al. 2018). It is believed that this is one reason why many kinds of nuts, if added to a person's diet, do not result in weight gain (Guarneiri and Cooper 2021). Effectively, many types of nuts, if eaten whole or in pieces, have a lower calorie density than the fat content would indicate.

We have laid out the essentials of a healthy diet in the previous paragraphs. Is it possible to eat this kind of diet and find it satisfying? We believe the answer is a clear "Yes!" In the chapter entitled "A Simple Diet," we mentioned the 2019 study by Hall et al. These investigators fed twenty people an unprocessed diet with a calorie density of about one calorie per gram, then an ultra-processed diet with about two calories per gram. Each diet was fed for two weeks, and which diet was given first was randomly decided. Subjects found the diets equally satisfying, though the unprocessed diet took about 29% longer to eat. The ultra-processed diet caused weight gain, and the unprocessed diet caused weight loss.

Thirty-six years earlier, before the coining of the phrase "ultra-processed," a similar study was done by Duncan et al. (1983). The goal was to understand the effects of calorie density on eating. Subjects were given a low-energy-density (LED) diet of 0.7 calories per gram or a high-energy-density (HED) diet at 1.5 calories per gram. There were ten obese and ten normal-weight subjects in the study. Half of each group were given the LED for five days followed by the HED for five days. The order was reversed for the remainder of each group. Subjects consumed about twice the number of calories on the HED diet compared to the LED diet. Overall, the two diets were found equally palatable, but the LED diet took 33% longer to consume. Interestingly, the obese and lean subjects did not differ in how many calories they consumed on either diet or how satisfied they were with the diets. These results demonstrate that LED diets can be palatable and successful in the short term.

If an LED diet can be palatable in the short term, then we think it is clear such a diet can be palatable in the long term. However, in practice, this has proved challenging. If there are both low-calorie and high-calorie items on the menu, studies show people will eat some low-calorie items but almost inevitably eat enough high-calorie items to make up for any decrease due to the low-calorie items. Much greater success comes when high-calorie items are not an option (Poppitt and Prentice 1996).

However, high-calorie options are ubiquitous in today's food environment. Because there is a strong correlation between the calorie density of foods and their fat content (Poppitt and Prentice 1996; Peters 2003), for practical purposes, an LED diet is a low-fat diet. One group that has succeeded in living long-term on an LED diet are subjects in the National Weight Control Registry (http://www.nwcr.ws/, [accessed June 27, 2022]). To become a member, one must have lost at least thirty pounds and maintained the loss for at least a year. The average weight loss is sixty-six pounds, and the average maintenance is five-and-a-half years.

In an analysis done in 2014 (Catenacci et all.), participants were found to eat a percentage of calories as fat that varied roughly between 25–33%. (Those maintaining the 25% level were found to be highly motivated.) This suggests that even for people who have had a weight problem, a diet with 33% of calories coming from fat is consistent with a normal or near-normal weight.

In another example, the Ole Study (Bray et al. 2002) recruited men who were overweight but otherwise healthy. The study was done to assess the efficacy of the fat substitute olestra, but our interest is in the two groups in the study who were not placed on olestra. One group, termed the "control group," were given a diet with 33% of calories from fat, and a second group, termed the "low-calorie group," were given a diet with 25% of calories from fat. The average weight loss in both these groups over the first three months was about equal: 3.3 kilograms. During the next six months the control group maintained their weight loss at about three kilograms, but the low-calorie group proceeded to gain back about half of what they had lost. They were apparently unable to endure the restriction and compensated by eating high-fat foods outside of the study protocol. We conclude that it is possible to follow an LED diet provided one does not restrict the fat too much. It is important to allow fat for the sake of palatability.

There are certain foods that are not health-promoting yet have great appeal. Dr. Neal Barnard names four foods that many people crave: meat, cheese, chocolate, and sugar (2018). While it is debated whether these and similar foods could be addicting (Greenberg and St. Peter 2021), our concern is their high-calorie density and ability to hijack any attempt to eat a healthy diet. It is generally agreed that they stimulate the same reward circuits in the brain that are stimulated by addicting drugs. Of course, these circuits are stimulated by anything we find rewarding.

The problem with these foods is they stimulate the reward circuits to an unnaturally high level. As a consequence, the reward circuits adjust themselves to this higher level of stimulation (Wallace and Fordahl 2021; Wang et al. 2002) and respond, though minimally, to the lower stimulation of healthy food (i.e., healthy food no longer provides much enjoyment). Just as a drug abuser's brain can recover through abstention, so can one recover from habitually eating an overly rich diet.

In recognition of this problem, Ellen White stated, "It will take time for the taste to recover from the abuses which it has received and to gain its natural tone. But perseverance in a self-denying course of eating and drinking will soon make plain, wholesome food palatable, and it will soon be eaten with greater satisfaction than the epicure enjoys over his rich dainties" (1923, p. 148). Regarding meat, she stated, "My position now is to let meat altogether alone. It will be hard for some to do this, as hard as for the rum drinker to forsake his dram; but they will be better for the change" (1938, p. 410).

White recommended against eating aged cheese in her day (see p. 368). We believe this was largely due to the risk of bovine tuberculosis and other milk-borne diseases, as pasteurization had not yet been introduced in the United States when her concerns were expressed. The problem of its digestion may also have been a concern. Regarding sugar, she stated "Far too much sugar is ordinarily used in food. Cakes, sweet puddings, pastries, jellies, jams, are active causes of indigestion" (p. 333).

While a healthy diet restricts indulgence in overly rich foods, it is not about deprivation. There are many meat substitutes on the market, which we enjoy eating perhaps once a week. We find it helpful to choose one with about ten grams of fat per serving, as digestion is much easier at that level. We find a cheese alternative made from cashew nuts and nutritional yeast is very tasty. We also occasionally use a little cheddar, mozzarella, or parmesan (milk-based) cheese to strengthen the flavor. Vegan cheese is also readily available, but it is not our favorite. Studies suggest that solid cheese can be difficult to digest (Drouin-Chartier et al. 2017; Guo et al. 2017; Peng et al. 2021); hence, we recommend using it more as a condiment than as a major ingredient in cooking.

While a healthy diet restricts indulgence in overly rich foods, it is not about deprivation.

We find vegetables tasty when well-cooked in a dash of olive oil and seasoned with a bit of salt and onions, garlic, or other herbs as desired. Instead of frying eggplant, we bake it. Likewise, French fries can be made by tossing potato slices with an olive oil and seasoning mixture, then baking them. Fresh fruit is a staple and provides wonderful flavors and textures. For special occasions, we enjoy fruit pie. We prefer an oil crust, but one must be careful, as an oil crust is rich; too much can be difficult to digest.

Food should be rewarding to eat; as vegetarians, we find it so. God gave the Israelites manna to eat. It is described thus: "the taste of it *was* like wafers *made* with honey" (Exod. 16:31); "The people went about and gathered *it,* ground *it* on millstones or beat *it* in the mortar, cooked *it* in pans, and made cakes of it; and its taste was like the taste of pastry prepared with oil" (Num. 11:8).

Ellen White opined, "To make food appetizing and at the same time simple and nourishing, requires skill; but it can be done. Cooks should know how to prepare simple food in a simple and healthful manner, and so that it will be found more palatable, as well as more wholesome, because of its simplicity" (1938, p. 257). "No one should adopt an impoverished diet. Many are debilitated from disease, and need nourishing, well cooked food. Health reformers, above all others, should be careful to avoid extremes. The body must have sufficient nourishment" (p. 91).

People are different and have different needs; some do well on one kind of food that seems harmful to others. Some have no trouble maintaining a healthy weight; others struggle to keep the pounds off. For those who struggle with their weight, there are some simple, proven strategies that can provide help. The first of these has the trending name "intermittent fasting." In essence, it does not involve fasting for long periods of time, but restriction is put on the time when food can be eaten (Rynders et al. 2019) during the week or during the day.

What we find particularly interesting is what has been termed "time-restricted eating" (TRE) and, more specifically, "early-time restricted eating" (eTRE). In TRE, one is allowed to eat in a time window of twelve or fewer hours each day (Adafer et al. 2020). In eTRE, the window for eating begins early in the day and generally ends by 3 p.m. (*Ibid.*; Sutton et al. 2018). Research shows that people who follow a TRE regimen eat 20% fewer calories and lose 3% of their body weight on average. These benefits are seen even in people who follow their usual diet (Adafer et al. 2020). There are also benefits in improved risk factors for cardiovascular disease. These benefits appear greater in those following eTRE and are seen even without weight loss (Sutton et al. 2018). Evidence suggests this is a consequence of better alignment of meal timing with the body's metabolic rhythms (Jakubowicz et al. 2021).

While eTRE seems to be a modern development, it is not. Dr. Charles D. Cupp, a graduate of Tulane University, practiced medicine in Texas from 1914–1977 and, from observation of his patients, proposed that weight problems were due to eating late in the day. He put his patients with weight concerns on a daily program of eating a large breakfast and either skipping supper or eating a light supper before 3 p.m. In any case, nothing was to be eaten after 3 p.m. Examination of his records reveal that those who followed his prescription lost weight, and type 2 diabetics who lost thirty pounds or more were cured of their diabetes (Carter and Brown 1985). Dr. Cupp credited his longevity to this program; he practiced medicine until age 96 and lived to be 104 years of age.

As it happens, eTRE has an even earlier history. Ellen White wrote, "I eat only two meals a day. But I do not think that the number of meals should be made a test. If there are those who are better in health when eating three meals, it is their privilege to have three. I choose two meals. For thirty-five years I have practiced the two-meal system" (1938, p. 178). She also had advice for those who eat three meals a day: "The practice of eating but two meals a day is generally found a benefit to health; yet under some circumstances, persons may require a third meal. This should, however, if taken at all, be very light, and of food most easily digested. Crackers—the English biscuit—or zwieback, and fruit, or cereal coffee, are the foods best suited for the evening meal" (p. 176).

White also recommended making breakfast the largest meal of the day: "It is the custom and order of society to take a slight breakfast. But this is not the best way to treat the stomach. At breakfast time the stomach is in a better condition to take care of more food than at the second or third meal of the day. The habit of eating a sparing breakfast and a large dinner is wrong. Make your breakfast correspond more nearly to the heartiest meal of the day" (p. 173). We believe most people with a weight problem would find eTRE very beneficial. Anyone on medication should work with their physician to make changes safely.

A second strategy to limit the amount of food eaten is to limit the number of different palatable foods offered at any one meal. Research on rodents has consistently shown that a diet offering a variety of highly palatable human foods leads to greater intake and weight gain than does a diet consisting of a single high-calorie food or a control diet of standard fare (Ferreira et al. 2018; Johnson et al. 2016; Leigh et al. 2019; Sampey et al. 2011; Zeeni et al. 2015). A recent review of human studies also concluded that "variety is a robust driver of food intake" (Embling et al. 2021).

Sensory-specific satiety is thought to be the basis for this phenomenon. Sensory-specific satiety is the concept that one tires of a particular taste fairly quickly, but this does not affect the desire for other tastes. Therefore, if you limit yourself to a few flavors at a meal, you will become satisfied before you overconsume. Sensory-specific satiety for simple flavors has been observed to function in obese and otherwise overweight people just as effectively as it does in normal-weight people (Brondel et al. 2007). This suggests reduced variety could help people with weight concerns.

Finally, a study of over 2,000 registrants in the National Weight Control Registry shows that these people who have maintained at least a 30-pound weight loss for an average of 6.1 years (all at least one year) eat a diet with reduced variety in all food categories (Raynor 2005). People with recent weight-loss success reduce the variety of foods they eat in the high-fat food categories, but those from the registry who have succeeded long-term partake of even less variety in the high-fat food categories on average (Raynor 2005).

Ellen White also gave instruction regarding the variety of foods served at a meal: "There should not be a great variety at any one meal, for this encourages overeating, and causes indigestion" (1938, p. 112); "There should not be many kinds at any one meal, but all meals should not be composed of the same kinds of food without variation. Food should be prepared with simplicity, yet with a nicety which will invite the appetite" (p. 110). She also gave specific instruction regarding the number of different foods to provide for a meal:

> "Do not have too great a variety at a meal; three or four dishes are a plenty. At the next meal you can have a change. The cook should tax her inventive powers to vary the dishes she prepares for the table, and the stomach should not be compelled to take the same kinds of food meal after meal....
>
> If your work is sedentary, take exercise every day, and at each meal eat only two or three kinds of simple food, taking no more of these than will satisfy the demands of hunger. (*Counsels on Diet and Foods*, pp. 109, 110)

A third strategy to limit the amount of food eaten is to take sufficient time for meals. Studies show a strong correlation between how fast a person eats and one's weight (Robinson et al. 2014; Ohkuma et al. 2015; Slyper 2021). This would be expected because food passing rapidly through the mouth has reduced time to provide sensory input, and this impairs sensory-specific satiety. Plant-based foods that are minimally processed generally require significant mastication, which is beneficial and can reduce intake (Slyper 2021; Miquel-Kergoat et al. 2015). Unfortunately, the modern food environment provides many highly or ultra-processed options that are soft and require little chewing. The conclusion is clear: Eat plant-based foods with little processing and with their natural fiber. Prefer solids over liquids and include some dry foods that require more chewing when practical. Finally, chew your food well. Take time to notice the flavors and enjoy them. Eating with friends can slow the process of eating and may provide benefit as well.

Ellen White emphasized both the importance of chewing and taking time to eat:

In order to secure healthy digestion, food should be eaten slowly. Those who wish to avoid dyspepsia, and those who realize their obligation to keep all their powers in a condition which will enable them to render the best service to God, will do well to remember this. If your time to eat is limited, do not bolt your food, but eat less, and masticate slowly. The benefit derived from food does not depend so much on the quantity eaten as on its thorough digestion; nor the gratification of taste so much on the amount of food swallowed as on the length of time it remains in the mouth. Those who are excited, anxious, or in a hurry, would do well not to eat until they have found rest or relief; for the vital powers, already severely taxed, cannot supply the necessary digestive fluids....

So much porridge eating is a mistake. The dry food that requires mastication is far preferable. The health food preparations are a blessing in this respect. Good brown bread and rolls, prepared in a simple manner, yet with painstaking effort, will be healthful. Bread should never have the slightest taint of sourness. It should be cooked until it is thoroughly done. Thus all softness and stickiness will be avoided. (*Counsels on Diet and Foods*, pp. 107, 318)

> *Some signals drive hunger and promote eating, while others alleviate hunger and suppress eating; all are designed to promote optimal health.*

The human appetite is an expression of very complicated interactions between the brain and the gut involving many hormones and neural connections (Ahima and Antwi 2008; Cifuentes and Acosta 2022). Some signals drive hunger and promote eating, while others alleviate hunger and suppress eating; all are designed to promote optimal health. It was White's teaching that if we would partake of food that is both healthy and palatable, it would require no extraordinary measures to maintain health and strength: "It is impossible to prescribe by weight the quantity of food which should be eaten. It is not advisable to follow this process, for by so doing the mind becomes self-centered. Eating and drinking become altogether too much a matter of thought" (1938, p. 108).

We interpret this statement to also rule out calorie counting as an approach to controlling intake. This assumes one is healthy and not dependent on medications to control glucose. "We always had something to say about the necessity of providing wholesome food and of preparing it simply, and yet making it so palatable and appetizing that those eating it would be satisfied" (p. 473). Palatable food provides a certain amount of stimulation for the pleasure centers of the brain. This, combined with gut neural and hormone signals, inform the brain that sufficient food has been ingested. "Eat according to your best judgment; and when you have asked the Lord to bless the food for the strengthening of your body, believe that He hears your prayer, and be at rest" (1905, p. 321).

CHAPTER 6

Obeying Your Body's Rhythms

The human organism is complex. The body consists of approximately 37 trillion cells of several hundred different types (Bianconi et al. 2013; Roy and Conroy 2018). The human brain consists of about 70 billion neurons (von Bartheld et al. 2016). Each human cell contains a copy of the roughly 3 billion bases of DNA that make up the human genome. The genome possesses about 20,000 basic genes that produce approximately 70,000 variant proteins because a single gene can frequently be used to make more than one protein (so-called "splice variants"). Once a protein is produced, the cell has several hundred ways it can be modified to change its function; consequently, there may be well over 1 million different forms of proteins with the potential for different chemical interactions (Aebersold et al. 2018). The body begins as a single cell having maximum potential, but as that cell divides, the successive generations of cells are programmed to particular cell types with limited potential in terms of the proteins they can make and how they can function. Certain cell types become programmed to become neurons; others, the liver; others, the kidney; still others, the heart, etc. Clearly, the human cell is capable of very sophisticated behavior.

While the human cell is capable of sophisticated behavior, a single human cell acting alone, because of its small size, can accomplish very little. Something must cause many cells to act together to produce a useful effect. Just as an army requires coordinated action to defeat the enemy, cells require coordinated action to produce the useful functions of the body. An army would not be able to accomplish its goals if the soldiers could not keep time. In the same way, cells need access to time signals to prepare for and act their part at the appropriate time. Fortunately, a benevolent Creator has provided us with genes that allow every cell to have a functioning clock. The clock consists of several genes and proteins that interact and cycle through the same set of reactions approximately every twenty-four hours.

A rough explanation of what goes on is that gene A produces protein A, which builds up its level until it turns on gene B to produce protein B. When protein B has reached a sufficient level, it acts to turn off gene A. There is also a mechanism in the cell that destroys both protein A and B. Since A is no longer being produced, its level falls. Once A is low enough, it no longer stimulates the production of B, and its level also begins to fall. When the level of B gets sufficiently low, we have completed the cycle, and the production of A is no longer inhibited; therefore, its production begins again. There are at least eight proteins and as many genes involved in the clock, which is designed to go through its cycle in just a little over twenty-four hours (Pacha and Sumova 2013; Patton and Hastings 2018). While it is important that our cells are equipped with clocks, this is only one step towards organization and concerted action.

For clocks to be ultimately useful, they need to not only keep time but the *same* time. In the human body, this is accomplished by the suprachiasmatic nuclei (SCN), located on either side of the brain just behind our eyes and above where the optic nerves cross. Each nucleus consists of about 10,000 neurons tightly coupled in their function by contacts between them so that their clocks keep the same time. This time would cycle at slightly over twenty-four hours, but our eyes have nerve cells that detect day and night, so they signal the SCN and nudge them to slightly speed up and cycle every twenty-four hours. The SCN are the master clocks for the body. Signals from them go out to the rest of the body to keep all its cells on the same twenty-four-hour cycle.

Since the SCN are not only located by but are part of the brain, they signal other parts of the brain through neural pathways. One of these neural pathways reaches the pineal gland near the back of the brain. It keeps its cells in time with the external environment so that it secretes the sleep hormone melatonin beginning in the evening and peaking in the middle of the night. This makes sense as melatonin makes one sleepy. If, for some reason, we need to be awake and doing something at night, our eyes sense the artificial light we are using and send signals to the pineal gland to slow the production of melatonin so we have a better chance of staying awake to accomplish whatever is needed. Of course, the body has many organs besides the pineal gland; all of them are kept on the same twenty-four-hour cycle by the SCN. In addition, each organ has its own clock with aspects specific to its function, but all these clocks are synchronized through communication with the SCN (Patton and Hastings 2018; Macchi and Bruce 2004; Peruri et al. 2022).

Another means of cellular control is through our conscious choices. With our brains, we make decisions to pick up a glass and take a drink, make a statement, read a book, or perhaps sit still and think about a problem. The nerves in our frontal cortex work to control other nerves in the motor cortex to control muscles when needed. However, nerves are expensive to run and maintain. Estimates place the brain at 2% of the body's weight while it receives 12% of the blood flow (Meng et al. 2015). Brain tissue uses energy over six times as fast as do other tissues per unit weight.

The body has more efficient mechanisms to communicate with most of its cells. Chemical messengers move with the flow of blood and are recognized by receptors on the surface of the cells they target or may enter the cell and interact directly with its structure. Most communication between our cells is of this chemical type and takes place without our conscious awareness. The body even uses amplification stages in important cases. The hypothalamus is a part of the brain located deep behind the eyes; it has nerves that make a small amount of several hormones that are known as releasing factors. The nerves secrete these factors near capillaries that carry the factors to the pituitary gland located just beneath the hypothalamus. The factors each target different cells in the pituitary, which cause the pituitary to release a more plentiful supply of a trophic hormone that circulates in the blood and causes a particular gland to secrete a hormone important in its function throughout the body.

For example, if we are under stress, our hypothalamus will secrete corticotropin releasing factor (CRF), which will be carried by the blood to the pituitary and cause it to secrete adrenocorticotropic hormone (ACTH). ACTH will then circulate in the blood and attach to receptors on cells in the adrenal glands and cause them to secrete the stress hormone cortisol that will in turn circulate throughout the body and act on all the cells to change their function to prepare for potentially stressful or harmful events.

While stress manifests itself through our hypothalamus to increase the production of CRF and ultimately the level of cortisol in our blood, the SCN also have an important influence on the same CRF-secreting neurons. The SCN are a part of the hypothalamus, and they exert a rhythmic signal that causes the secretion of CRF in a recurring pattern within a twenty-four-hour cycle. The effect of stress, when it happens, is just superimposed on this rhythm. The SCN also control the body's temperature within a twenty-four-hour cycle.

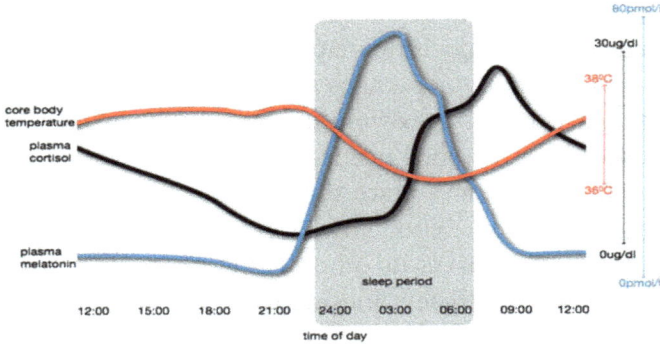

Figure 1. The normal synchronous relationships between sleep and day time activity and varying levels of cortisol, melatonin, and body temperature (Hicki et al. 2013). Creative Commons Atribution 2.0 Generic.

The blood levels of melatonin and cortisol and the core body temperature over a twenty-four-hour period are shown in Figure 1. In the figure, the grey area represents sleep time. The figure shows sleeping at the optimal time in relationship to melatonin levels. Remember, melatonin makes you feel sleepy. Notice the body temperature in relation to sleep. It is believed that body temperature directly affects our alertness level; therefore, we would be most alert when our body temperature was highest (excluding a process such as a fever). However, as we are awake and active during the day, sleep debt builds up. When it reaches its peak in the evening, we fall asleep in spite of our body temperature (Borbely et al. 2016). During the night as we sleep, our sleep debt is being paid, but we do not awaken because our body temperature falls, and we become less alert. When the sleep debt is sufficiently paid, we awaken in the early morning.

If we have had a good night's sleep, we awaken refreshed and ready for another day after seven or eight hours of restorative sleep. Notice the cortisol level peaks in the early morning. Cortisol acts throughout the body to mobilize energy stores and prepare the body for intense activity if needed. It is anti-inflammatory and inhibits protein synthesis, both of which are required in healing (Riad et al. 2002). Cortisol reaches its lowest level between about 9 p.m. and 3 a.m. This is the optimal time for synthesizing proteins to rebuild tissues and for inflammation to promote healing. Sleep generally begins during this period; typically, slow-wave or deep sleep happens early in the night. With slow-wave sleep also comes the secretion of growth hormone by the pituitary gland. This promotes healing as well (Takahashi et al. 1968; Wilmore 1999).

The rhythmic change in cortisol, melatonin, and body temperature just described is but the tip of the iceberg. It has been estimated that 80% of all proteins produced in the body are created in a circadian rhythmic pattern in some tissue so that their levels tend to be low in the daytime and high at night or vice versa. It may help to understand at least part of the reason for this if you think of your automobile. Most of the time, you use it for transportation, but several times a year, it is necessary to get it serviced and possibly repaired. We are quite comfortable with the fact that we cannot use the car for transportation at the time it is being serviced and repaired. These are two distinct phases of an automobile's existence.

In the same way, our cells have important functions in our bodies to help us reach our life's goals, but they also need time for repair and restoration. Indeed, cells suffer from damage to their DNA and the other structures within them; however, mechanisms in our cells perform the needed repairs. Intriguing studies in fruit flies, mice, and zebrafish show that double-stranded breaks in the DNA of neurons occur preferentially when the organism is awake and are repaired during sleep (Bellesi et al. 2016; Zada et al. 2019). There are also mechanisms within cells to perform a process called "autophagy" ("self-eating"). This process has several forms, one of which is also known as "programmed cell death" or "apoptosis," in which the whole cell breaks down its own substance and neatly packages its substance in membrane-bound droplets ready for the cells of the immune system to remove.

We cannot use the car while it is being repaired. In the same way our cells also need time for repair and restoration.

Other forms of autophagy simply target damaged parts of a cell (and recycle them) or even individual damaged proteins or no-longer-needed proteins (D'Arcy 2019; Saha et al. 2018). In macroautophagy, the cell surrounds an organelle by a double-layered membrane known as an "autophagosome." The autophagosome is then joined to a lysosome that digests its contents and recycles them for reuse by the cell. Studies in the fruit fly have shown that macroautophagy is governed by a circadian rhythm. If the feeding time of flies is restricted in a particular pattern, nighttime macroautophagy is enhanced. As a result, flies have a lengthened life span and health span. Switching day for night in these experiments does not prolong life or health (Ulgherait et al. 2021; Yin and Klionsky 2022). Fruit flies sleep at night while mice sleep during the day. Studies in mice show that mice preferentially experience macroautophagy in the daytime (Juste et al. 2021; Ma et al. 2011).

Another form of autophagy is known as "chaperone mediated autophagy" (CMA). In CMA, a protein known as a "chaperone" attaches to a protein to be recycled and moves it into a lysosome, where it is digested and its constituent amino acids are made available for reuse. Studies in mice have shown that CMA is largely circadian in expression with different proteins targeted for removal at different times of the day. This programming is different for different organs (Juste et al. 2021; Ma et al. 2011; Kaushik et al. 2022). The detailed play and counterplay of protein creation and destruction largely in circadian rhythms, specific to each organ and cell type, governed by the master clock, and all working together to produce life, has called forth the word "astonishing" (Patton and Hastings 2018). While much more remains to be learned, one conclusion is compelling: There are preferred times for different activities.

Our circadian rhythms are determined by the day-and-night cycle. It is difficult to change this unless you live in a cave and spend most of your time there (Boivin et al. 2022). Consequently, for most of us, the optimal time to sleep is at night, when our melatonin level is high. People who work nightshifts are a prime example of the results of sleeping at a time not synchronized with the body's rhythms. Studies show that most events in the body continue to happen with the same circadian rhythms on the same time schedule, but with a reduced amplitude. The melatonin level still peaks at night, the cortisol level peaks in the early morning, and the temperature peaks in the late evening, but the peaks are not as high, and the low points are not as low. Individual cells appear to be working correctly, but they are not acting together at the same level. Conflicting light signals and the unusual timing of meals and sleep have this effect, which causes shifts in metabolism that are not optimal (Boivin et al. 2022).

As a consequence, nightshift workers experience a higher level of obesity, metabolic syndrome, type 2 diabetes, and heart disease as well as some cancers (Boivin et al. 2022). While nightshift work is likely to take a significant toll on one's health, studies of sleep show that sleep difficulties are problematic for health regardless of their origin. Much epidemiological data indicate a strong connection between too little sleep (<5–6 hours/night) or too much sleep (>8–9 hours/night) and the risk of type 2 diabetes, heart disease, and strokes, as well as an increased risk of cancer (Cappuccio et al. 2010; Fernandez-Mendoza et al. 2019). These data are further corroborated by a Mendelian Randomization study of over 2 million people, which draws similar conclusions (Jia et al. 2022). Mendelian Randomization is a statistical technique that provides evidence of causality; in this case, sleep problems cause health problems.

Given the importance of sleep, what can we do to ensure we sleep well? One important prescription is to go to bed at the same time in the evening and get up at the same time in the morning. If you follow such a routine, your mind and body will become accustomed to the routine. You will fall asleep more easily and wake up more ready for the day (Dement and Vaughan 1999, pp. 425, 426). Studies show that irregularity in sleeping is strongly associated with delayed sleep or evening chronotype, daytime sleep and sleepiness, as well as increased cardiometabolic risk (Lunsford-Avery et al. 2018).

Interestingly, greater sleep irregularity was not associated with less sleep. Sleep was just more fragmented and more in the daytime. Thus, staying up late in an effort to accomplish more does not succeed in extending the time to accomplish one's goals. Assuming one is going to sleep on a regular schedule, should one go to bed early or late? The evening chronotype has been studied and found to be associated with a higher risk of metabolic syndrome and insulin resistance as well as a less active lifestyle (Vera et al. 2018). This study found some evidence of a genetic predisposition to be an evening chronotype, but no evidence that this genetic predisposition extended to the adverse health consequences has been found.

More recently, a much larger Mendelian Randomization study of the morning chronotype has been published (Jones et al. 2019). In this study, it was found that the 5% of people with the most morning predictive genes slept on average 25 minutes earlier than did the 5% with the least morning predictive genes (presumably, mostly evening types). Similar attempts to show a relationship between sleep duration and sleep quality were unsuccessful. Likewise, the presence of morning predictive genes provided no information about the likelihood of type 2 diabetes or a person's BMI. These data are important as they argue strongly that we should not blame our genes for any tendency we may have to stay up to very late hours rather than sleep.

Our sleep debt needs to build up for about sixteen hours to cause us to fall asleep easily. If we regularly get up at 5 a.m., we will be ready to fall asleep at about 9 p.m. when our circadian alertness has reached its peak (body temperature in Figure 1). Then our body temperature or circadian alertness will be falling throughout our sleep period and help keep us asleep until we have rested for seven-to-eight hours. Other important factors in getting good sleep are daily exercise, avoiding meals or stimulants near bedtime, a dark, cool, quiet room, and a comfortable bed (CDC, https://1ref.us/byb07, [accessed April 19, 2024]).

Another important activity that affects our circadian rhythms is eating. It is known that the hormone ghrelin stimulates hunger and generally rises shortly before a meal. An experiment on six young, healthy humans was carried out to measure their blood ghrelin levels every twenty minutes for a period of twenty-four hours (Natalucci et al. 2005). They were told they would not eat during this time with no possibility of seeing or smelling food. Blood levels of ghrelin peaked about a half hour before their usual mealtimes and decreased from that point until near the next meal. This provides evidence that ghrelin is under a strong circadian influence.

Much experimental evidence in rodents and humans indicates that the enzymes of digestion and the molecules that assist in transporting nutrients into the bloodstream are all under circadian control and created in anticipation of food intake (Pacha and Sumova 2013; Martchenko et al. 2020; Segers and Depoortere 2021). This makes sense, as it takes cells a significant period to create these substances. The body learns from the timing of meals and will even alter the rhythm of clocks in the gastrointestinal tract to accommodate those engaged in nightshift work who eat at times that are not optimal. The message is clear: Regularity in meal timing is an advantage to the organism, for without regularity, the body cannot be prepared for nutrient intake.

Assuming one eats at regular times, what times are optimal for health? Several lines of evidence point to morning as the best time for a meal. First, our cells are more sensitive to insulin in the morning. A good breakfast seems to reinforce our circadian rhythms and has a beneficial effect on blood sugar and insulin levels even at later meals (Jakubowicz et al. 2021; Richter et al. 2020). Second, the best evidence suggests that those who skip breakfast are less physically active than those who have a good breakfast (Clayton and James 2016). Finally, those who eat a good breakfast have a decreased appetite and less desire for high-fat meals (Jakubowicz et al. 2021; Beaulieu et al. 2020). Some evidence suggests those who eat a large breakfast find more pleasure in eating than do those who eat a large dinner (Versteeg et al. 2017).

We believe the evidence strongly supports a large breakfast as the best way to begin the day. The question is then, How long should one wait before eating again? Four large observational studies are unanimous in finding that those who eat more than three times a day, whether extra meals or snacking, experience increased weight and/or disease risk (Kahleova et al. 2017; Mekary et al. 2013; Mekary et al. 2012; Neuhouser et al. 2020). One large observational study found that those who eat three meals per day between two and four-and-a-half hours apart have a higher risk of dying than do those whose inter-meal intervals are between four-and-a-half and five-and-a-half hours. (Observational studies simply observe what people are doing and the consequences.)

The interesting thing about all five of these studies is that none of them were focused on questions of body weight or obesity at the time of data collection. A large amount of data was simply collected from all who entered the studies with the expectation that it would be useful. Several smaller observational studies of meal frequency or timing with a focus on questions of weight and weight control have not agreed with these larger studies. The discrepancy is explained by reporting bias; people who are overweight are embarrassed to give correct details about their food intake. As often as 50% of the time, they do not (Howarth et al. 2007; MoCrory and Campbell 2011).

Randomized controlled trials (RCTs) are helpful here because they randomly assign people to behave in one way or another and then observe the difference in consequences of the different behaviors. Such trials guard against explanations for the consequences that have eluded investigators. RCTs add strength to one's conclusions. RCTs show that those eating the same number of calories in six meals per day, compared with three meals per day, are hungrier throughout the day (Jakubowicz et al. 2019; Ohkawara et al. 2013). One of these trials involved diabetics given diets estimated to be 500 calories below the number needed to maintain weight (i.e., diets designed for weight loss).

Those in the three-meal sector ate a large breakfast, moderate lunch, and small supper (roughly 700, 600, and 200 calories, respectively). Those in the six-meal sector ate meals more equal in calories (350, 350, and 350 calories), with each meal followed two-to-three hours later by a 150-calorie snack. Those in the three-meal sector lost weight, had their insulin reduced, and experienced better blood sugar control than did those in the six-meal sector. They also saw higher-amplitude circadian rhythms (Jakubowicz et al. 2019).

In another RCT, all participants were healthy young men. Some were control participants who were given their usual diet. The remainder were given a diet with 40% more calories than their usual diet. Half of them ate three meals a day and simply added the extra calories to their meals. The remainder ate their extra calories as snacks two-to-three hours after their usual meals. Weight gain was the same in the two high-calorie groups, but those eating six times a day saw a significant fat build-up in their liver compared to the control group, while those on the three-meal program did not (Koopman et al. 2014). It was concluded that those eating more than three times a day may be putting themselves at risk for fatty liver disease. We believe the evidence supports no more than three meals a day and preferably at least five hours apart.

Ellen White gave instructions regarding regularity in one's habits that largely agree with the research we have examined regarding sleeping and eating:

> Make it [a] habit not to sit up after nine o'clock. Every light should be extinguished. This turning night into day is a wretched, health-destroying habit, and this reading much by brain workers, up to the sleeping hours, is very injurious to health. It calls the blood to the brain and then there is restlessness and wakefulness, and the precious sleep that should rest the body does not come when desired.
>
> It is needful to take care of the body and to study its needs and preserve it from unnecessary exposure. It is a sin to be ignorant of how to care for the wants of this habitation God has given us. Especially should brain workers begin to be soothed and not in any way excited as they draw nigh their hours for sleep. Let the blood be attracted from the brain by some kind of exercise, if need be. Let not the brain be taxed even to read, and, of course, not to put forth literary effort. (*Daughters of God*, p. 177)
>
> I know from the testimonies given me from time to time for brain workers, that sleep is worth far more before than after midnight. Two hours' good sleep before twelve o'clock is worth more than four hours after twelve o'clock." (*Manuscript Releases*, vol. 7, p. 224)
>
> Our God is a God of order, and He desires that His children shall *will* to bring themselves into order and under His discipline. Would it not be better, therefore, to break up this habit of turning night into day, and the fresh hours of the morning into night? If the youth would form habits of regularity and order, they would improve in health, in spirits, in memory, and in disposition. (*Child Guidance*, p. 112)
>
> Diligent study is not the principal cause of the breaking down of the mental powers. The main cause is improper diet, irregular meals, and a lack of physical exercise. Irregular hours for eating and sleeping sap the brain forces. (*Counsel on Diet and Foods*, p. 395)

In 1993, my youngest son was living with us and taking computer science at a local university. He seemed to be struggling with the schoolwork, and I noticed his habits were not regular. I offered him $1,000 if he would try a regular time for meals and get to sleep by 10 p.m. every night for a quarter. Since he was saving money to buy a car, he took me up on the deal. It proved very beneficial for him; he finished his degree in computer science and has had a good-paying job in the field since graduation, including regular bonuses in recent years. A recent study of Harvard University students found that those who are the most regular in their sleep habits sleep no longer than those who are most irregular, but those with the regular sleep have better academic performance (Phillips et al. 2017).

Regarding meals, Ellen White gave further instruction:

When my wife and I were married, she was accustomed to sleeping extra hours on weekends, but every Monday, she would suffer a migraine headache.

> The habit of eating a sparing breakfast and a large dinner is wrong. Make your breakfast correspond more nearly to the heartiest meal of the day.…
>
> If a third meal be eaten at all, it should be light, and several hours before going to bed.…
>
> After the regular meal is eaten, the stomach should be allowed to rest for five hours. Not a particle of food should be introduced into the stomach till the next meal.…
>
> Regularity in eating is of vital importance. There should be a specified time for each meal. (*Counsels on Diet and Foods*, pp. 173, 174, 179)

When my wife and I were married, she was accustomed to sleeping extra hours on weekends, but every Monday, she would suffer a migraine headache. I told her we needed to make a change. I would fix breakfast every day if she would get up at a regular time seven days a week and have breakfast with me. She agreed, and her Monday migraine headaches disappeared. She still suffered from migraine headaches on occasion, but not on Monday mornings. Regularity in eating and sleeping are known preventive measures that all can take with many additional health benefits as well.

CHAPTER 7

Exercise and Your Health

If we think of our bodies as an assemblage of organs, then Paul's statement expresses a certain truth: "But God composed the body ... that there should be no schism in the body, but *that* the members should have the same care for one another. And if one member suffers, all the members suffer with *it;* or if one member is honored, all the members rejoice with *it*" (1 Corinthians 12:24–26). As our knowledge of physiology has grown, it has become increasingly clear how our organs depend on each other for their ability to do their tasks.

For the kidneys to do their work, there must be sufficient blood pressure to move the blood through the kidneys' vascular system. If the kidneys sense too low a blood pressure, they secrete an enzyme called "renin." To have its effect, renin must convert angiotensinogen, which is made in the liver, to angiotensin I. Angiotensin I must then be converted to angiotensin II in the lung and kidneys. Angiotensin II acts on the blood vessels to constrict them and raise the blood pressure. It also acts on the adrenal glands to cause the production of the steroid hormone aldosterone, which can cause the retention of salt by the kidneys as well as on the brain to make one thirsty and on the posterior pituitary gland to produce more antidiuretic hormone to cause the retention of water by the kidneys (Fountain et al. 2023). Thus, by multiple mechanisms involving multiple other organs, the blood pressure rises, and the kidneys are helped to do their work.

Perhaps surprisingly, our muscles have the potential for many interactions with the other organs in our bodies. It has been estimated that our muscles secrete over 200 substances through which they communicate with our fat tissue, liver, pancreas, bones, and brain, among others. These substances modulate the energy flowing to the muscles from our fat stores and the food we eat, stimulate the growth and health of the nerves and blood vessels that interact with the muscles, and generally contribute to our health by decreasing inflammation throughout the body (Legård and Pedersen 2019).

If we can be healthier through exercise, then it is important to ask how much and what kind of exercise is beneficial and what is known of the benefits. One of the key guidelines for Americans put forward by the US Government is "For substantial health benefits, adults should do at least 150 minutes to 300 minutes a week of moderate-intensity, or 75 minutes to 150 minutes a week of vigorous-intensity aerobic physical activity, or an equivalent combination of moderate- and vigorous-intensity aerobic activity. Preferably, aerobic activity should be spread throughout the week" (USDHHS 2018).

To understand the meaning of these exercise guidelines, we must understand what moderate-intensity and vigorous-intensity exercise mean. A person who sits quietly is said to burn energy at the rate of one metabolic equivalent (1 MET), generally measured to be 3.5 milliliters of oxygen used per kilogram of body tissue per minute. If one is actively exercising, then oxygen is being burned more rapidly; this is measured in multiples of 1 MET. If one is burning oxygen three times as fast as when sitting quietly, then we say one is burning oxygen at 3 METs. Three METs is the threshold for moderate physical activity. If one is burning oxygen at 6 METs, then one has reached the level of vigorous physical activity. It is helpful to have an idea of the kinds of activities that require a moderate or vigorous level of effort. See a sample of such activities in Table 1. The guidelines call for moderate activity (at least 3 METs) for 2.5 hours per week or vigorous activity (at least 6 METs) for 1.25 hours per week. Mathematically, 3 METs x 2.5 hours = 6 METs x 1.25 hours = 7.5 MET-hours per week.

Table 1. A selection of common activities and the level of effort required in METs (Ainsworth et al. 1993).

Moderate activity	METs	Vigorous Activity	METs
Bicycling, leisurely	4	Bicycling, 10 mph	6
Vacuuming	3.5	Chopping wood	6
Mopping	3.5	Shoveling snow	6
Raking lawn	4.3	Hand sawing	7
Walking, 3 mph	3.3	Jogging	7
Bowling	3	Basketball, game	8
Playing frisbee	3	Jumping rope	10

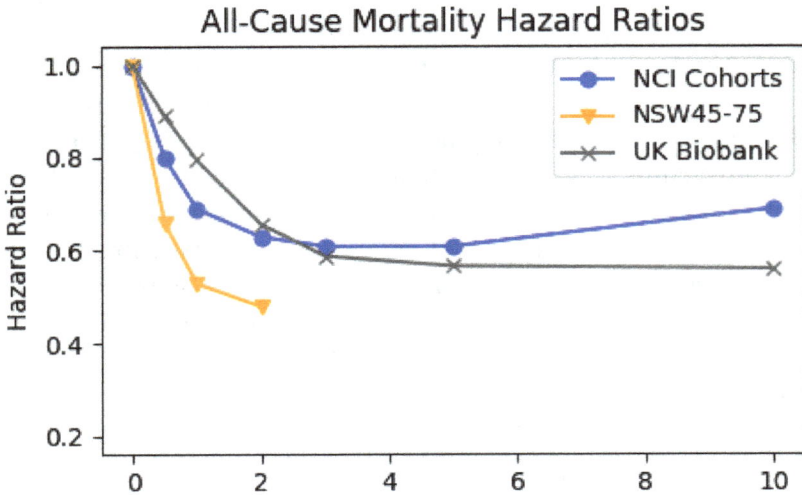

Figure 2. All-cause mortality hazard ratios for three large groups of people as a function of exercise quantity. One unit along the x-axis means 7.5 MET hours/week for the blue and orange curves, but 2000 steps/day for the grey curve.

Fortunately, a large, pooled analysis of over 600,000 people published by the US National Cancer Institute addresses the benefits to be realized by meeting these exercise guidelines (Arem et al. 2015). Results are shown in Figure 2, specifically, the blue curve. The 1.0 in the upper left corner of the graph represents the reference point (i.e., those who do not exercise). Note that all the points to the right on all the curves are below 1.0 in value representing that they have a lower risk of death because they do exercise. The point on the blue curve at 0.5 units to the right represents those who exercise some but did not reach the guideline level of 150 minutes of moderate intensity exercise per week. Even they have a relative risk of 0.8, meaning they are 20% less likely to die of any cause then those who achieve no moderate intensity exercise in a given week.

The points at 1 unit and 2 units to the right are those who achieve at least the level of exercise and at least twice the level of exercise prescribed by the guidelines. Note that these points have relative risks of 0.69 and 0.63, respectively; the risk does not get significantly lower than that along the blue curve. The risk even appears to move slightly up at 10 times the guideline-recommended level of exercise, but there is too little data to be sure the risk has increased (Arem et al. 2015).

The orange curve is constructed the same way and with the same meaning as is the blue curve, but based on just over 204,000 residents of New South Wales, Australia (Gebel et al. 2015). We do not have an explanation for the lower hazard ratios seen on the orange curve, but one observation seems pertinent. The second, third, and fourth points on the orange curve seem to produce about the same shape as the second, third, and fourth points on the blue curve. The big difference is between the first (reference point) and the second points on the two curves. This would be explained if the reference group for the orange curve is composed of people much more likely to die than are those in the reference group for the blue curve. This would force all the other points on the orange curve to have low hazard ratios, as is seen in the graph.

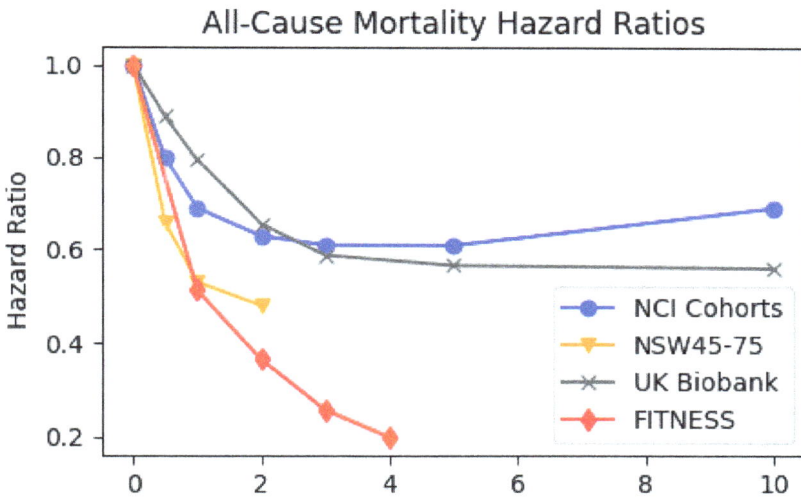

Figure 3. This figure is the same as figure 2 except for the addition of the red curve which represents the hazard ratio for death from any cause as a function of aerobic fitness. The reference point at height 1 represents the least fit individuals and successive points to the right represent increasingly fit individuals.

While 7.5 MET-hours per week is a useful exercise goal, it does not fit everyone's style. Many now monitor their steps per day. The value of steps per day is the subject of the grey curve in 2. This curve is based on a study of 78,500 UK Biobank participants (del Pozo et al. 2022). Each unit to the right on this curve represents an additional 2,000 steps/day. The authors state they saw no additional benefit in more than 10,000 steps/day. The hazard ratio at 10,000 steps/day is 0.57, which is a significant 43% reduction in risk of death compared with those who take few steps in a given day.

We may ask, Why does the grey curve initially not show as much benefit as do the blue or orange curves? The answer is that one may take thousands of steps each day without engaging in any moderate or vigorous exercise, but the evidence strongly supports an added health benefit when our exercise is more vigorous. In the UK Biobank study, those who took steps at a higher rate had a lower hazard ratio compared with the same number of steps taken more slowly (del Pozo et al. 2022). Experiments show that a step rate of at least 100 steps/minute corresponds to a moderate exercise level; at least 130 steps/minute, a vigorous exercise level (Tudor-Locke et al. 2021). Likewise, in the New South Wales study, those who engaged in some vigorous exercise experienced a 9% reduction in the risk of death, while those who obtained at least 30% vigorous exercise experienced a 13% advantage (Gebel et al. 2015).

While measuring the amount we exercise can provide an estimate of the health benefit we obtain, there is a more incisive way to measure the benefits of exercise. Aerobic fitness or the maximal number of METs one can reach on an exercise treadmill has been found to correlate strongly with the risk of death from any cause. Data from a large study by the Cleveland Clinic (Mandsager et al. 2018) on risk of all-cause mortality as a function of fitness are contained in Table 2 and displayed as the red curve in Figure 3. The authors of this study comment that there seems to be no limit to the benefit of aerobic fitness in terms of decreasing the risk of death. This contrasts with quantity of exercise, which seems to reach a lower limit in hazard ratio beyond which more exercise does not benefit, as illustrated by the blue, orange, and grey curves in the figure. This seems reasonable, as the exercise we perform will require us to reach a certain number of METs. Just because we carry it on for a longer time may not confer an ability to reach a higher number of METs.

Table 2. All-cause mortality hazard ratios for groups defined by percentile level of fitness within a population of 122,007 consecutive patients referred for exercise treadmill testing (Mandsager et al. 2018).

Hazard Ratio	Fitness Percentile	Average Group Fitness
1.0	<25th low	6.1 METs
0.51	25th –49th below average	8.2 METs
0.36	50th –74th above average	9.6 METs
0.26	75th –97.6th high	11.4 METs
0.20	97.7th ≤ elite	13.8 METs

While high aerobic fitness confers a low mortality risk, this does not prove that improving one's fitness will provide such a benefit. However, as a rule, people only have a high aerobic fitness level if they have trained to achieve it, which is sufficient reason to recommend exercise as an approach to lowering mortality risk (Mandsager et al. 2018; Myers et al. 2002). Assuming we would like to improve our aerobic fitness, a reasonable approach is reduced-exertion high-intensity interval training (REHIT) developed in the recent past (Metcalfe et al. 2015; Vollaard and Metcalfe 2017; Vollaard et al. 2017). The REHIT protocol is quite simple:

- Warm up for 3 minutes.
- Do a 20-second all-out sprint.
- Recover for 3 minutes.
- Do a 20-second all-out sprint.
- Cool down for 3 minutes.

This protocol is typically carried out on an exercise bike, though we have also found it useful on an elliptical machine. In order to effectively perform the exercise, one must be sure the exercise machine is set at a high enough difficulty level that the all-out sprint really prompts maximal effort. Experiments have shown this approach to be more effective than continuous moderate-intensity exercise is in increasing aerobic fitness and much more time efficient (Cuddy et al. 2019; Ruffino et al. 2017; Thomas et al. 2020). One can hope for about a 10% increase in aerobic fitness and a corresponding 12–15% decrease in mortality risk (Myers et al. 2002; Cuddy et al. 2019; Lee et al. 2011).

Attempts to decrease the amount of exercise involved in REHIT have shown it is ineffective if one only does a single all-out sprint (Songsorn et al. 2016) per session; it also loses effectiveness if one decreases the sprint time from twenty seconds to ten or fewer (Haines et al. 2021; Nalcakan et al. 2018). Interestingly, two REHIT sessions per week seem to be as effective as are three or more (Thomas et al. 2020). However, the data show that REHIT is only effective in producing a clinically meaningful increase in aerobic fitness in about half of those who attempt it (Metcalfe and Vollaard 2021). For those who are not accustomed to regular vigorous physical exercise, we recommend they obtain clearance from their doctors before attempting REHIT. A personal trainer may also be helpful.

Another aspect of exercise that is embraced by The Physical Activity Guidelines for Americans is strength training. "Adults should also do muscle-strengthening activities of moderate or greater intensity and that involve all major muscle groups on 2 or more days a week, as these activities provide additional health benefits" (USDHHS 2018). We know that strength peaks at about age 25 in humans and proceeds to decline at a rate of from 1–2.5% per year (Degens 2019). At their peak, men generally have 1.5–2 times the strength of women, but the decline happens at about the same rate percentage-wise. As a consequence, women will reach a level of weakness causing disability in their late seventies, whereas men will reach the same level in their early nineties unless an effort is made to prevent this (Degens 2019). Even in older people who engage in habitual running for exercise, it has been found that the leg muscles decrease in strength at a rate of 3–5% per year (Marcell et al. 2014). This result also suggests the rate of strength decline accelerates with age.

> *We know that strength peaks at about age 25 in humans and proceeds to decline at a rate of from 1–2.5% per year.*

Strength training seems to be most beneficial in older people with whom too much aerobic exercise seems to hasten the decline in strength. It has been found even in advanced age that strength training can be very effective in increasing strength. An eighty-year-old who engages in strength training may have the strength of a sixty-year-old who does not (Aagaard et al. 2010). While strengthening the muscles through weight training can provide real benefits, the bad news is that the benefits are limited and will decline with age as already described (Aagaard et al. 2010). There is also evidence that in older people, too much weight training can eliminate any benefit. Something under an hour a week seems to provide all the benefit possible, which is estimated to be about a 12% reduction in all-cause mortality (Patel et al. 2020). Additional support for this low-volume approach is provided by experiments showing that three thirteen-minute sessions per week in which each exercise is done at one set per session was sufficient to maintain strength; more sets per session did not increase strength (Schoenfeld et al. 2019).

Ellen White was a proponent of the benefits of exercise, especially of walking:

Those whose habits are sedentary should, when the weather will permit, exercise in the open air every day, summer or winter. Walking is preferable to riding or driving, for it brings more of the muscles into exercise. The lungs are forced into healthy action, since it is impossible to walk briskly without inflating them.

Such exercise would in many cases be better for the health than medicine. (*The Ministry of Healing*, p. 240)

There is no exercise that can take the place of walking. By it the circulation of the blood is greatly improved.... Walking, in all cases where it is possible, is the best remedy for diseased bodies, because in this exercise all of the organs of the body are brought into use....

Morning exercise, in walking in the free invigorating air of heaven, ... is the surest safe-guard against colds, coughs, congestions of the brain and lungs, ... and a hundred other diseases. (*Healthful Living*, pp. 129, 210)

While White highly recommended walking, she recognized the value of other forms of exercise:

Exercise, to be of decided advantage to you, should be systematized, and brought to bear upon the debilitated organs that they may become strengthened by use....

God designed that the living machinery should be in daily activity; for in this activity or motion is its preserving power.

By active exercise in the open air every day the liver, kidneys, and lungs also will be strengthened to perform their work. (*Healthful Living*, pp. 128, 131)

The first sentence in the quote above seems consistent with what we would recognize today as physical therapy, but White recommended exercise in the form of useful labor as sufficient in many cases:

Useful employment would bring into exercise the enfeebled muscles, enliven the stagnant blood, and the entire system would be invigorated to overcome bad conditions....

When useful labor is combined with study, there is no need of gymnastic exercises; and much more benefit is derived from work performed in the open air than from indoor exercise. (*Healthful Living*, pp. 46, 128)

We highly recommend walking for many reasons. Walking is generally safe if the environment is safe. Walking outdoors exposes you to fresh air and sunshine with their added benefits. Walking only requires some good shoes as equipment. In the summer, you will need protection from the hot sun. In the winter, the arms and legs need to be kept warm to encourage the free circulation of the blood. If you are not used to walking, begin slowly with only five minutes, then gradually increase the time in five-minute increments until you can walk thirty minutes.

For those who struggle with weight issues, many find it helpful to walk an hour a day. If you are pressed for time and can tolerate it, you can walk at a fast pace. Remember, 100 steps per minute gets you into the moderate-intensity exercise category, for which everyone should aim, while 130 steps per minute or more constitutes vigorous exercise, which has special benefits in terms of aerobic fitness.

If you are approaching the senior years but new to strength training and feel you could benefit from it, we recommend the little book Growing Stronger - Strength Training for Older Adults (https://1ref.us/byb17). It is freely downloadable and will give you a great starting point.

CHAPTER 8

Health Beliefs and Their Consequences

We know our beliefs affect our actions, which in turn can have health consequences. However, we may be less aware of how our beliefs can affect our health without any conscious action on our part. As an example, consider the case of internal mammary artery blockage as therapy for coronary artery disease. This surgery was performed in the late 1950s because it was reasoned that blockage of the blood flowing through the main internal mammary artery would lead to a greater flow to the heart muscle. This would take place through one of its small upstream branches, which supplied a portion of the heart muscle, much like blocking the flow in one branch of a creek may cause water to back up and flow in a new channel that is not blocked.

Those performing the surgery were gratified to find that many patients thus treated described a very significant improvement in symptoms. However, some questioned whether such an intervention involving so small an artery to the heart muscle could really be of significant benefit. Therefore, experiments were undertaken in which two groups of patients were treated. In one such study, eight patients received standard internal mammary ligation (blocking), and nine patients received sham surgery in which the patient underwent anesthesia and the chest wall was opened, but no ligation was carried out. The results were of great interest. Even though the physicians performing the surgery could not be blinded to what they had done, the patients were very effectively blinded.

Six months following surgery, both groups of patients reported modest increases in exercise tolerance and a decrease in the use of nitroglycerin: 34% in the ligated group, and 42% in the sham group. One patient who received sham surgery experienced outstanding benefits. Prior to the treatment, after four minutes of exercise, he would experience chest pain, and marked electrocardiogram (EKG) changes indicated ischemia of the heart muscle. Six weeks after the treatment, he could exercise for ten minutes without any pain or EKG changes (Beecher 1961; Miller 2012).

A second study by different surgeons led to the same conclusion: Sham surgery was just as effective as actual ligation was. In another example of the same phenomenon, Lown (1977) followed a forty-year-old angina patient with serial exercise testing. It was found that the patient experienced chest pain and ST segment depression on the EKG tracing consistently after forty-four crossings (two steps up followed by two steps down). During the tests, the physician reported the number of crossings audibly, and the patient noted the relationship between the count and the sensation of pain. There followed a series of six stress tests; in four of them, the physician falsified the count and stated the count as forty-four when it was only thirty-two.

In each of the six tests, the patient experienced the expected chest pain and ST depression when the count of forty-four was announced. On the seventh test, the count was falsified again at forty-four, but the patient recognized that the count was incorrect and experienced no pain or ST depression. Significantly, ST depression on the EKG tracing reflects a change in the physiology of cardiac muscle, which is not generally under conscious control. About a month after the last exercise test, the patient died of a heart attack.

The examples just presented of patients with angina who improved after sham surgery, as well as the patient who had chest pain (angina) when he thought he had exercised more than he had, yet with no chest pain at the same exercise level when he was not deceived, are representative of what is known as the placebo effect. An excellent definition of the placebo effect follows: "A placebo effect is a change in a patient's illness attributable to the symbolic import of a treatment rather than a specific pharmacologic or physiological property" (Turner et al. 1994). In other words, a placebo effect is a consequence of a medication or treatment that cannot be explained based on physical or chemical principles without appealing to the state of mind of the patient. Arguably, the heart patients who had sham surgery would not have improved had they not believed they would be improved by the surgery; likewise, the heart patient who experienced chest pain at thirty-two crossings would not have experienced the pain had he not believed he would. In these cases, the effect was the result of a state of mind. In the case when a placebo effect is harmful, it has come to be known as a negative placebo effect or "nocebo" effect (Kennedy 1961).

The placebo effect is recognized as a ubiquitous phenomenon throughout the practice of medicine. Virtually any treatment a doctor may prescribe will involve a placebo effect at some level. While not all patients will experience a placebo effect, as a general rule, 30% of patients are likely to feel benefited by the placebo effect; however, the figure can be much higher depending on the intervention (Turner et al. 1994). Some important factors in determining the strength of the placebo effect are listed below (Beecher 1961; Turner et al. 1994; Geier 1994; Kelkar and Ross 1994; Straus and von Ammon Cavanaugh 1996; Tudor Hart and Dieppe 1996):

1. The patient's level of stress or need.

2. The patient's level of hope or expectation of help from the treatment.

   a. The level of control the patient perceives over his disease as credited to the placebo.

   b. The level of belief and enthusiasm of the physician and other healthcare workers who interact with the patient.

   c. Expense and impressiveness of the treatment.

   d. Culturally conditioned expectations of what is effective treatment (symbolism).

Examples of 2c are the observation that surgery is a powerful placebo and a shot is more effective than a pill is (Beecher 1961; Turner et al. 1994). Examples of 2d are the observations that pill color is important for the placebo effect, a greater number of pills is perceived as more effective, and a capsule produces a greater effect than a tablet does (Buckalew and Coffield 1982; Hussain and Ahad 1970; Sallis and Buckalew 1984; Schapira et al. 1970). A study of a new antihypertensive medication about which the investigators were very enthusiastic provides a good illustration of 2b. When the investigators were subsequently told that the medication was of similar strength to current medications but not told which patients were receiving the medication and which were receiving placebo, it was found that those on the medication continued to show the lower blood pressures, but in both the new medication and placebo groups, blood pressures went up markedly (Shapiro et al. 1954).

One can find many other impressive examples of the placebo effect. Much of the data that corroborate the placebo effect comes from studies with a control group, a treatment group, and patients who are aware of these two groups. The patients do not know in which group they have been placed, but ethical considerations require that they be informed and consent to be in a study in which they know they may receive only a placebo. This tends to reduce the patient's expectations of benefit and hence the magnitude of any placebo effect that is seen.

To demonstrate this fact, researchers who had previously conducted a study of patients with tinnitus (ringing in the ears) restudied some of their patients. The original study had been a comparison of placebo (saline) injection with lidocaine (a local anesthetic). They contacted twenty-five of the patients who had received placebo treatment in this study. Twenty agreed to a trial of lidocaine to see if it would actually help them. The investigators, however, gave them shots of saline again. The patients now believed they were definitely receiving lidocaine. Forty percent responded with an improvement in their symptoms, and most of these had not responded to the placebo in the previous trial (Duckert and Rees 1984).

As already mentioned, the placebo effect can work in a negative direction as well as a positive direction. Results depend on what the patient is led to expect. In a study of the effects of instructions on patients' gastrointestinal responses, it was found that when patients were told a pill would increase stomach motility, have no effect, or decrease motility—where in all cases the pill given was the same and only contained the magnet used to measure stomach motility—the patients' responses significantly fulfilled expectations (Sternbach 1964). In a study of asthmatic patients given a placebo (salt water), those told the treatment would cause bronchodilation experienced bronchodilation, and those told the treatment would cause bronchoconstriction experienced bronchoconstriction. In those given a true bronchodilator medication, the measured bronchodilation was twice as great in those led to expect bronchodilation as in those told to expect bronchoconstriction (Luparello et al. 1970).

In a study of thirty-four unselected college students, more than two thirds reported mild headaches when told that a nonexistent electric current was passing through electrodes attached to their heads, which might cause a headache. While no control group was reported, only one of the people who experienced a headache had a history of more than one headache a month. Thus, it seems clear that we are dealing with a very marked nocebo response (Schweiger and Parducci 1981).

Thomas (1987) reports studying a group of 200 of his patients who had no definite signs of disease and for which no diagnosis could be made. The patients were randomized into positive and negative groups. Those in the positive group were given a diagnosis and told they would be better in a few days. Those in the negative group were told by the doctor that he was uncertain of what was wrong with them. Two weeks later, 64% of the positive group but only 39% of the negative group reported that their conditions had improved. He concluded that since most such conditions improve without treatment within two weeks, the low improvement rate in the negative group represents a nocebo response.

The Truth About Medical Treatments. Much of the history of medical practice is a history of treatments that were actually harmful to the patient! As late as the early part of the twentieth century, surgeons believed that simply cutting open a person's abdomen and then sewing it closed again was beneficial for patients with tuberculosis of the lining of the abdominal cavity—likewise for women with pelvic infections (Beecher 1961). In the same era, surgeons removed people's colons in an attempt to cure epilepsy.

When it was realized that such treatments could have no effect on the cause of the disease involved, these practices stopped. What seemed to be benefits were only placebo responses.

Much of the history of medical practice is a history of treatments that were actually harmful to the patient!

Because surgery carries risks and has a mortality rate, these surgical treatments were, in general, harmful and could be deadly. The fact that some patients might feel improved for a time is not sufficient justification for these risks. Physicians subscribe to the Hippocratic Oath, which forbids the giving of deadly medicine to anyone. Furthermore, it is not considered ethical to lie to a patient or charge money for a treatment that is useless, much less harmful. Unfortunately, not all physicians are ethical in their behavior. Some will stoop to virtually any device or deception to make money. As a protection for the public, in 1962, the US Food and Drug Administration put into effect a regulation that all medicines must be proven safe and effective. It is estimated that thousands of drugs were removed from the market at that time (McMahon 1994).

One of the important contributions of an understanding of the placebo effect has been in the design of valid experiments to determine the effectiveness of medical treatments. The placebo effect alone will make any form of treatment that is not overtly harmful appear to have some level of effectiveness. Therefore, it is not sufficient to simply give a certain number of patients a particular treatment and see if some reasonable fraction find the treatment helpful. In most such cases, even if there is no specific effect of the treatment on the disease, at least 30% and sometimes as high as

80% of the patients will report improvements in symptoms (Straus and von Ammon Cavanaugh 1996).

The recognition of this fact has given rise to placebo-controlled trials in which patients are randomized into two groups. One group is designated the control group and receives an inactive or placebo treatment. The second group receives the prospective treatment. If this test treatment benefits patients significantly more often than does the placebo treatment as ascertained by appropriate statistical testing, the test treatment is considered effective. Actually, matters are a little more complicated. It is necessary that the patients in the two groups do not know which treatment they are receiving. Such a knowledge would preclude those receiving the placebo treatment from being able to believe in the efficacy of their treatment, and they would be unlikely to feel benefited from doing something they considered equivalent to doing nothing. Thus, the patients must be blinded to what kind of treatment they are receiving.

Furthermore, if the physicians or other caregivers know which treatment the patients are receiving, they may be more reassuring to those receiving the test treatment or, in some other subtle way, inspire confidence in the test treatment as opposed to the placebo treatment. Because the level of confidence of a patient in his or her physician and the physician communicating expectations to the patient are important factors in the placebo effect, such an occurrence would destroy the validity of the test. It is therefore necessary that not only the patient but also the physician and other healthcare workers dealing with the patient be blinded to which treatment the patient is receiving. Thus, ideally, trials are double-blind, randomized, and controlled. If these conditions can be met, one can, with considerable confidence, ascertain the true value of a treatment as compared with a placebo.

Controlled, randomized, double-blind trials have been the key to a scientific approach to medicine. Without this approach, it would be impossible to separate truth from fiction in many areas of medical practice and research. The need for such trials is largely the result of the placebo effect, which seems like an annoyance in imposing such a demanding approach on efforts to arrive at truth. On the other hand, the placebo effect is often very positive in its contribution to the patient's well-being, even when that patient is taking medication that has been proven effective in its own right. McMahon (1994) may have been right when he concluded, "the placebo has made probably the single most important contribution to modern therapeutics of any drug."

The Truth About Ourselves. We can learn an important lesson about ourselves in the story of the placebo: We are easily deceived regarding what is good or bad for us. If we are convinced that some medication or treatment will benefit us and we try it, we are likely to experience a placebo effect. The natural next step is to interpret this experienced benefit as clear evidence of the efficacy of the medication or treatment. Likewise, if we are convinced that something will be harmful to us and we try it, we are likely to experience a nocebo effect. The natural conclusion is then to take this as proof that it is inherently bad for us. When we confirm our beliefs or suspicions in this manner, we are more convinced of their correctness; therefore, the stage is set to strengthen the effect.

By the strength of the placebo effect's confirmation, people can become believers in error and the performance of things definitely detrimental to themselves. As an example, we cite the tragic case of Eben Byers (Macklis 1993). Byers, a prominent New York socialite and steel magnate, died in 1932 of a mysterious illness. At the time of his death, he was fifty-two years old. He had been a handsome, athletic man and former US amateur golf champion. When death came, we are told, "He weighed just 92 pounds. His face … had been disfigured by a series of last-ditch operations that had removed most of his jaw and part of his skull in a vain attempt to stop the destruction of bone. His marrow and kidneys had failed, giving his skin a sallow, ghastly cast."

Upon examination, physicians learned he had died of radium poisoning. Due to persistent pain secondary to an injury that was not responsive to other treatment, his private physician had suggested that Byers try the patent medicine Radithor. The manufacturer claimed Radithor was a cure for over 150 different maladies, including dyspepsia, high blood pressure, and impotence. It is estimated that during the next five years or so, Byers drank over 1,000 bottles of this highly radioactive substance. "He told friends that he felt invigorated and rejuvenated. So satisfied was he with the results that he sent cases to his friends, colleagues and female acquaintances and even fed some of the expensive potion to his racehorses" (Macklis 1993). When the deadly effects of Radithor became known, many people came forward with their personal supply of the medicine. "Among them was Mayor James J. Walker of New York City, who at first refused to give up his radioactive rejuvenator because, he said, it made him feel so good." Today, the dangers of radiation are widely known and appreciated, so we are not so tempted to trust our imaginations when scientific data gives unquestioned support to the contrary.

As a young person, I read a book entitled *Body, Mind, and Sugar* by Abrahamson and Pezet, which taught that most human illness and even crime was due to episodes of low blood sugar. I became a believer that I suffered from hypoglycemia and felt this was a problem that plagued me until I became a medical student. When I made my complaint known to the student health service, I was invited to present myself for a blood test when I experienced symptoms. I did so, and the results did not confirm the diagnosis. I suddenly no longer believed I had the problem. The scientific evidence to the contrary was enough for me.

I had also come to believe, from false literature on the subject, that my stomach did not produce enough acid and I would be helped by taking hydrochloric acid tablets, which could be purchased at the health food store where my mother worked at the time. Indeed, I felt better when I took the pills and significant indigestion when I did not take them. When I got to the subject of pharmacology in medical school, the professor pointed out that some people take hydrochloric acid tablets because they think that will help digestion, but the amount of acid in the pills is minuscule in comparison to what the stomach produces. I stopped taking the pills and felt no ill effects. Knowledge had cured me of another disease. I had not realized that for years, I had been practicing an absurdity. Truly, the words of Solomon are full of wisdom: "The simple believes every word, but the prudent considers well his steps" (Prov. 14:15).

While the placebo effect can lead one to believe in and practice things that are useless or even harmful, the nocebo effect can cause us to avoid things that would be good for us if we only believed so. As a young person, I once became quite ill with vomiting when engaging in work that was very physically taxing. After that, I thought such exertion was harmful and avoided it if possible. I even noticed I felt bad when engaging in any vigorous exertion, which seemed to confirm my suspicion. When I arrived at medical school, I still believed this was one of my problems. In a class on psychiatric illness, I was taught that some people had a neurotic fear of exercise, which was termed "neurasthenia." I was not interested in having any psychiatric diagnosis other than normal. I forthwith began a morning program of running and suffered no ill effects, though this is a very vigorous form of exertion.

Approximately three fourths of Americans do not get the daily exercise needed for optimal health (CDC, https://1ref.us/byb08, August 2022). While we do not know how many Americans refrain from exercise because they fear ill effects, it is estimated that in the USA, somewhere between

836,000 and 2.5 million people suffer from something called "Chronic Fatigue Syndrome" (CFS) (CDC, https://1ref.us/byb09, [last reviewed January 28, 2021]). The cause is unknown, and no test is diagnostic for the condition. The diagnosis is based on history and symptoms described by the patient. As a rule, patients experience excessive fatigue from exercising; fear of exercise is prominent. There is no proven cure.

The most promising approach to treatment of which we are aware is based on the PACE trial results (White et al. 2011; Sharpe et al. 2022). The PACE trial compared Cognitive Behavioral Therapy (CBT) and Graded Exercise Therapy (GET) with the usual approaches to therapy and concluded that CBT and GET were more effective. A subsequent analysis of the data pointed to fear-avoidance behavior (e.g., "I am afraid that I will make my symptoms worse if I exercise") and its amelioration as a key mediator of the benefit coming from CBT and GET (Chalder 2015). Basically, this says the nocebo effect resulting from the fear of exercise is an important part of the disease process. Despite its logic, this is not widely accepted in the field of medicine. The search continues for some explanation that will make sense of the very heterogeneous group of patients who carry the CFS diagnosis (Deumer et al. 2021).

In this context, it is important to note that studies have not revealed any muscular defect that would make exercise challenging (Gibson et al. 1993) or any cardiovascular defect that would preclude vigorous exercise on the part of CFS patients (Cook et al. 2022; Sisto et al. 1996). CFS patients were modestly less efficient than control participants were in eliminating the CO_2 generated during exercise (Cook et al. 2022). According to a study of people enrolled in the Framingham Heart Study, such decreased ventilatory efficiency is associated with risk factors for cardiovascular disease such as diabetes, high BMI, smoking, and decreased physical activity. In virtually all such cases, increased exercise would reduce the cardiovascular risk (Del Pozo et al. 2022; Harris et al. 2019; Ho et al. 2022; Yu et al. 2003).

Ellen White had something to say to those who feared to exercise in her day:

> Disease is sometimes produced, and is often greatly aggravated, by the imagination. Many are lifelong invalids who might be well if they only thought so. Many imagine that every slight exposure will cause illness, and the evil effect is produced because it is expected. Many die from disease the cause of which is wholly imaginary. (*The Ministry of Healing*, p. 241)

The key clause here is "the evil effect is produced because it is expected," which is a concise description of the nocebo effect.

Thousands are sick and dying around us who might get well and live if they would; but their imagination holds them. They fear that they will be made worse if they labor or exercise, when this is just the change they need to make them well. Without this they never can improve. They should exercise the power of the will, rise above their aches and debility, engage in useful employment, and forget that they have aching backs, sides, lungs, and heads. Neglecting to exercise the entire body, or a portion of it, will bring on morbid conditions. (White, *Medical Ministry*, p. 105)

> *It can be difficult to break away from the strength of habits and fears that bind us to practices that are detrimental to our health. Ellen White models a successful approach.*

It can be difficult to break away from the strength of habits and fears that bind us to practices that are detrimental to our health. Ellen White, in her own experience, models a successful approach. She had been a meat eater but became convinced she should give up meat for the sake of improved health:

When making these changes in my diet, I refused to yield to taste, and let that govern me. Shall that stand in the way of my securing greater strength, that I may therewith glorify my Lord? Shall that stand in my way for a moment? Never!

I suffered keen hunger, I was a great meat eater. But when faint, I placed my arms across my stomach, and said, "I will not taste a morsel. I will eat simple food, or I will not eat at all." Bread was distasteful to me. I could seldom eat a piece as large as a dollar. Some things in the reform I could get along with very well; but when I came to the bread, I was especially set against it. When I made these changes, I had a special battle to fight. The first two or three meals, I could not eat. I said to my stomach, "You may wait until you can eat bread." In a little while I could eat bread, and graham bread, too. This I could not eat before; but now it tastes good, and I have had no loss of appetite. (*Counsels on Diet and Foods*, p. 483)

Vinegar is a known irritant that can cause serious injury to the lining cells of the stomach (Nakao et al. 2014; Okabe and Amagase 2005). White's experience in giving up vinegar was remarkable:

> For weeks I was very sick; but I kept saying over and over, The Lord knows all about it. If I die, I die; but I will not yield to this desire. The struggle continued, and I was sorely afflicted for many weeks. All thought that it was impossible for me to live. You may be sure we sought the Lord very earnestly. The most fervent prayers were offered for my recovery. I continued to resist the desire for vinegar, and at last I conquered. Now I have no inclination to taste anything of the kind. This experience has been of great value to me in many ways. I obtained a complete victory. (*Counsels on Diet and Foods*, p. 485)

Many appeal to experience to justify their habits, but the validity of experience seems little understood. White had this to say about the nature of trustworthy experience:

> That which many term experience is not experience at all; it is simply habit, or mere indulgence, blindly and frequently ignorantly followed, with a firm, set determination, and without intelligent thought or inquiry relative to the laws at work in the accomplishment of the result.
>
> Real experience is a variety of careful experiments made with the mind freed from prejudice and uncontrolled by previously established opinions and habits. The results are marked with careful solicitude and an anxious desire to learn, to improve, and to reform on every habit that is not in harmony with physical and moral laws. The idea of others' gainsaying what you have learned by experience seems to you to be folly and even cruelty itself. But there are more errors received and firmly retained from false ideas of experience than from any other cause, for the reason that what is generally termed experience is not experience at all; because there has never been a fair trial by actual experiment and thorough investigation, with a knowledge of the principle involved in the action. (*Testimonies for the Church*, vol. 3, pp. 68, 69)

I have no doubt that if Ellen White were alive today, she would welcome the randomized, controlled, double-blind clinical trial as a gift from God to better attain a knowledge of scientific truth.

Chapter 9

Substance Use

We begin this chapter with a few basic facts about how your brain and nerves function. Your brain is made up of billions of cells, the role of which is to transmit signals. A signal may travel from your finger up your arm, into your spinal cord, up to your brainstem, and then to the sensory part of your cortex. To do so, it must travel through several nerve cells in succession. Signals also travel many pathways within the brain from one nerve cell to another.

Nerve cells have long, thin branches of two types. Dendrites are shorter and bring incoming signals to the cell body. Axons are longer and carry signals away from the cell body to meet a dendrite on the next cell body in the signal's path. The axon does not physically touch the dendrite to transmit its signal. Rather, there is a space between the axon and dendrite called a "synaptic cleft." When the signal on the axon arrives at the synaptic cleft, the signal causes the end of the axon to secrete a chemical neurotransmitter. This chemical diffuses across the synaptic cleft and becomes attached to another chemical called a "receptor" on the dendrite.

When sufficient chemicals are bound to receptors on the dendrite, this stimulates a signal in the dendrite. In order to limit the time the neurotransmitter is in the cleft stimulating the dendrite, there is often also a transporter molecule that binds the neurotransmitter and moves it back into the axon for reuse. In this way, the signal on the axon bridges the gap between the two nerve cells. There are many different chemical neurotransmitters, each with its own receptor and transporter to which it will bind. Different neurotransmitters are used in different parts of the brain. Some neurotransmitters that have attracted much study are glutamate, serotonin, dopamine, norepinephrine, and acetylcholine. Medications that block the reuptake of serotonin and norepinephrine have been found useful in the treatment of some cases of depression. The substances cocaine, methamphetamine, amphetamine, and ecstasy block the reuptake of dopamine and are frequently implicated as drugs of abuse.

To say drugs like cocaine, methamphetamine, heroin, and tobacco are health-destroying hardly needs a defense. We all know these are substances to avoid in the interest of health. Given this fact, we will limit our discussion of them. However, these substances have been studied rather intensely to learn how they addict. What has been learned, we believe, has broad application in understanding human behavior. All these substances and many others can stimulate pleasurable sensations in the brain. What they have in common is the ability to raise the level of the neurotransmitter dopamine (DA) in the brain. They do not all act in the same manner, but the common thread is the elevation of dopamine by one mechanism or another.

The pleasurable sensations as reported by humans have been found to correlate with elevated levels of DA in select parts of the brain. The higher the level of dopamine, the more pleasurable the reported sensation. The involved parts of the brain are commonly referred to as the reward circuits. In particular, they are known as the mesolimbic, mesocortical, and nigrostriatal DA circuits (Volkow et al. 2002). The mesolimbic pathway includes the nucleus accumbens, amygdala, and hippocampus and is thought to be strongly involved in the reward experience, reward memories, and learning. The nigrostriatal pathway includes the substantia nigra and dorsal striatum and is believed to be involved with habit formation, as seen in chronic drug use. The mesocortical pathway includes the prefrontal cortex, orbitofrontal cortex, and cingulate gyrus. Evidence suggests these are involved in judgment, motivation, and self-control (Volkow et al. 2002; Feltenstein et al. 2021). Based on current understanding, important events in addiction to drugs of abuse can be outlined:

- Drugs of abuse cause an artificial elevation of DA in the reward circuits that is substantially above that obtained from natural reinforcers such as healthy food (Volkow et al. 2002; Feltenstein et al. 2021; Volkow et al. 2007; Volkow et al. 2011; Volkow et al. 2017).

- Continued use of drugs of abuse with continued significant elevation of DA leads to down regulation of dopamine D2 receptors (DAD2R) and even a decrease in the level of DA resulting from a given drug dose (Volkow et al. 2002; Volkow et al. 2007; Volkow et al. 2011; Volkow et al. 2017). This has two important consequences:

- ○ Natural, healthy reinforcers are now too weak to bring significant pleasure (Volkow et al. 2011; Martin-Soelch et al. 2001; Cowan and Devine 2008).

- ○ Even the drug may no longer bring pleasure and is only used to try to experience a modicum of normality (Volkow et al. 2011; Volkow and Fowler 2000).

- • Over time, the downregulated (i.e., decreased) stimulation in the mesocortical pathways leads to lowered activity in the cortical regions critical to judgment and inhibitory control. As a result, discontinuing drug use becomes much more of a challenge (Volkow et al. 2002; Feltenstein et al. 2021; Volkow et al. 2007; Volkow et al. 2011; Volkow et al. 2017).

By using radioactive molecules that bind to dopamine D2 receptors, it is possible to show that the reduction in receptors in the striatal regions of the brain is on the order of 10–20% in cocaine, methamphetamine, heroin, and alcohol addiction when compared with non-addicted controls (Volkow et al. 2002). Further studies show that the lower the D2 receptors in the striatal regions of the brain, the lower the rate of glucose metabolism in the frontal cortical regions when the subjects are not experiencing the effects of the addictive substance (Volkow et al. 2002; Volkow et al. 2007; Volkow et al. 2011). A low rate of glucose metabolism indicates decreased cellular activity in the vital frontal lobes and suggests an explanation for the impaired judgment so prevalent in addiction (Volkow et al. 2002; Feltenstein et al. 2021).

Food satisfies all the criteria for addiction that originally led to the US Surgeon General's report concluding that cigarettes are addicting.

Several studies have reported a decrease in cortical grey matter volume in those who abuse drugs as compared with non-addicts (Cowan et al. 2003; Daumann et al. 2011; Ersche et al. 2011; Grodin et al. 2021; Matochik et al. 2003; Thompson et al. 2004). This gives evidence of what could be permanent damage to the cortical grey matter. One report provides evidence that video gaming addiction can provide a dopamine stimulus comparable with hard drugs and lead to similar structural brain damage (Weinstein et al. 2017).

While food addiction is not a widely accepted concept, food does stimulate the same reward circuits on which drugs of abuse act. It has been convincingly argued that food satisfies all the criteria for addiction that originally led to the US Surgeon General's 1988 report concluding that cigarettes are addicting (Gearhardt and DiFeliceantonio 2023). It has been observed that those who are obese suffer from a rate of tobacco use double that of the non-obese and have a more difficult time quitting (Ely and Wetherill 2022). This is hypothesized to be because food and nicotine act on the same reward pathways. The same reasoning has been used to suggest a relationship between obesity and other forms of substance abuse (Vanbuskirk and Potenza 2010).

Those suffering drug addiction may eat little; however, on coming off the drug, individuals describe indulging in high-fat or high-sugar foods as a temporary way of coping (Cowan and Devine 2008; Chavez and Rigg 2020). Perhaps the most impressive evidence for food as an addictive substance is the decrease in dopamine D2 receptors inversely proportional to the BMI, observed in morbidly obese people, and the impact this must have on frontal lobe function (Volkow et al. 2017; Wang et al. 2002; Wang et al. 2001; Zhang et al. 2022). One may ask how food could be addicting when it does not cause the high dopamine levels in the synaptic cleft that is seen with abused drugs. It is hypothesized that lower dopamine levels are made up for by increased frequency of stimulation (Volkow et al. 2017).

Coffee is a stimulant that has purported health benefits; it is claimed that 3.35% of healthy-life years lost to death or disability would be saved if all adults drank one cup of coffee per day; it would increase to 6% if all consumers drank three cups per day (Doepker et al. 2022; Crippa et al. 2014; Grosso et al. 2016). Two things need to be remembered concerning these conclusions. First, they are based on observational data rather than randomized controlled trials and do not constitute a proof of the conclusions. Second, no one has been able to explain why coffee should confer such a benefit. It has been suggested that antioxidants in coffee could provide the health benefits, but proof is lacking (Doepker et al. 2022; Crippa et al. 2014; Grosso et al. 2016). The caffeine in coffee has been a concern and does constitute a risk in some situations (Rodak et al. 2021); however, a dose of 400 milligrams per day or fewer is considered generally safe for adults (Wikoff et al. 2017).

While the studies just quoted seem to give coffee a clean bill of health, some modern methods of examining the brain are beginning to raise questions. It has been found that the offspring of women who drank up to three cups of coffee per day while pregnant are at an increased risk for obesity and behavioral problems. A recent study showed that even at the presumed safe prenatal dose of up to two cups of coffee per day for the mother, her nine-to-eleven-year-old offspring will likely have brain structural changes, including "greater posterior and lower frontal cortical thickness and altered parietooccipital sulcal depth" (Zhang et al. 2022). The significance of these findings is yet to be understood.

Clearer are the results of three recent studies showing that the volume of grey matter is decreased in those who habitually use coffee (Kang et al. 2022; Lin et al. 2021; Zheng and Niu 2022). Two of these studies are Mendelian randomization studies involving large numbers of subjects and implying that coffee consumption is responsible for decreased grey matter volume (Kang et al. 2022; Zheng and Niu 2022). One study also examines cereal grain intake and finds it has the opposite effect and increases grey matter volume (Kang et al. 2022). Test scores on several cognitive tasks were found to correlate positively with grey matter volume (Kang et al. 2022).

These findings on grey matter volume remind one of the decreased cortical thickness observed in the brains of those addicted to drugs. Since caffeine is not a stimulant comparable to hard drugs such as cocaine or methamphetamines, it may seem surprising that it should have such an effect. However, caffeine is metabolized to paraxanthine, which also has a significant stimulant effect and is metabolized more slowly so that people who drink coffee daily will have elevated levels of paraxanthine in their blood 24/7 (Lin et al. 2021). We suggest that the constant stimulation due to paraxanthine may explain how coffee can have its effect on grey matter volume.

In Ellen White's day (1827–1915), the options for addiction were fewer but still readily available. She warned of these and also included a warning regarding tea and coffee:

> The sure effect of narcotics and unnatural stimulants as tea, coffee, tobacco, beer and wine, is to enfeeble and degrade the physical nature, and lower the tone of intellect and morals. Any unnatural excitement of the nervous system affects the brain nerve power. We have a work before us to educate the people, line upon line, and precept upon precept. We must teach them that health and even life is endangered by the use of stimulants which excite the exhausted energies to unnatural, spasmodic action. ("The Necessity for Immediate Action," *Sanitarium Announcement*, January 1, 1900)

Tea ... enters into the circulation and gradually impairs the energy of body and mind. It stimulates, excites, and quickens the motion of the living machinery, forcing it to unnatural action, and thus gives the tea drinker the impression that it is doing him great service, imparting to him strength. This is a mistake.

Tea draws upon the strength of the nerves and leaves them greatly weakened. When its influence is gone and the increased action caused by its use is abated, then what is the result? Languor and debility corresponding to the artificial vivacity the tea imparted.... Coffee is a hurtful indulgence. It temporarily excites the mind, ... but the aftereffect is exhaustion, prostration, paralysis of the mental, moral, and physical powers. The mind becomes enervated, and unless through determined effort the habit is overcome, the activity of the brain is permanently lessened. (*Temperance*, pp. 76, 77)

The use of flesh as food was also a concern for White, as it could be addicting and have a negative impact on the mind.

When the use of flesh food is discontinued, there is often a sense of weakness, a lack of vigor. Many urge this as evidence that flesh food is essential; but it is because foods of this class are stimulating, because they fever the blood and excite the nerves, that they are so missed. Some will find it as difficult to leave off flesh eating as it is for the drunkard to give up his dram; but they will be the better for the change. (*The Ministry of Healing*, p. 316)

It is impossible for those who make free use of flesh meats to have an unclouded brain and an active intellect. (*Counsels on Diet and Foods*, p. 389)

If meat can be addicting (Barnard 2018), this suggests it can overstimulate the dopamine D2 receptors in the brain. This would then lead to down regulation of these receptors, just like in drug addiction, and have a negative impact on mental function. White was not concerned about mental function only but also spiritual impact. Addiction not only blunts the mental powers but also the spiritual perceptions. With this, Scripture agrees: "Harlotry, wine, and new wine enslave the heart" (Hosea 4:11); "Beloved, I beg *you* as sojourners and pilgrims, abstain from fleshly lusts which war against the soul" (1 Peter 2:11).

CHAPTER 10

Dealing with Your Mind

On their web page, the American Psychiatric Association gives the following brief definition of mental illnesses: "Mental illnesses are health conditions involving changes in emotion, thinking or behavior (or a combination of these). Mental illnesses can be associated with distress and/or problems functioning in social, work or family activities" (https://1ref.us/byb15, [accessed April 19, 2024]). We could loosely paraphrase this definition to say mental illness is abnormal thinking that causes distress or seriously effects one's ability to cope with life. Emotions and behavior almost always follow as a consequence of thoughts. This is true of most major conditions considered mental illnesses, such as schizophrenia (SCZ), bipolar disorder (BPD), major depressive disorder (MDD), obsessive compulsive disorder (OCD), autism spectrum disorder (ASD), attention-deficit/hyperactivity disorder (ADHD), and anorexia nervosa (AN).

In the current understanding, mental disorders are defined by descriptive collections of symptoms. This has led to some difficulty because observation shows that close to half of those who satisfy the criteria for one diagnosis also satisfy the criteria for at least one additional diagnosis (Kessler et al. 2005; Taylor et al. 2023). Such patients present a diagnostic and treatment dilemma and experience a more severe course of illness (Taylor et al. 2023). In a further twist, large studies show that those who have received one diagnosis of a mental illness frequently receive one or more other diagnoses at later stages in their lives (Caspi et al. 2020; Plana-Ripoll et al. 2019). These facts call into question the current classification of mental illness and have led to a search for a deeper understanding (Caspi and Moffitt 2018; Lee et al. 2021; Smoller 2013; Su et al. 2022).

Studies of family relationships have proven helpful in revealing that the same genetic alterations that predispose to one mental illness in a family increase the likelihood of other mental illnesses in blood-related family members. For example, the Taiwan National Health Insurance (NHI) program insures over 99% of Taiwan's residents and collects information on diagnoses as well as family relationships. A study of SCZ, BPD, MDD, ASD, and ADHD revealed 431,887 cases in the NHI database (23 million patients). These were compared with control patients without one of these mental disorders. Results showed that if a patient had SCZ, then his or her first-degree relatives had a risk factor for SCZ 6.4 times that of first-degree relatives of controls; BPD, 3.3; MDD, 2.0; ASD, 2.7; and ADHD, 1.8 times (Su et al. 2022). In fact, any one of these five conditions increased the risk in first-degree relatives of any of these conditions by a factor of at least 1.7 with one exception—the sole exception: If a patient is diagnosed with MDD, his or her first-degree relatives have a slightly lower risk of 0.9 of being diagnosed with SCZ compared to relatives of control group participants. This indicates common genetic factors underlying all these conditions. Besides the Taiwan NHI, a sibling study of the Swedish population also came to similar conclusions (Pettersson et al. 2016).

Because of the human genome project and the increasing availability of genetic sequence information from large numbers of people, it is now possible to do comparative studies of the genetic material of people with a particular disease versus people without that disease. Such studies are called GWAS (genome-wide association studies). They allow investigators to identify gene alterations (variants) that have a high likelihood of contributing to the occurrence of a disease. GWAS applied to the study of mental illness has confirmed not only that mental illness in general has a strong genetic component, but also different forms of mental illness often share many of the same genetic variants. This has led investigators to categorize several mental illnesses into three overlapping groups, where there is a major sharing of genetics within each group. These groups are:

- SCZ, BPD, MDD (mood and psychotic disorders)
- MDD, ASD, TS (Tourette's syndrome), ADHD (early neuro developmental disorders)
- TS, AN, OCD (compulsive/perfectionistic behaviors) (Lee et al. 2021).

Further study of the genes that mental illnesses share, as well as those not shared, holds out the hope of a much clearer understanding of pathological processes underlying mental illness; however, much work remains to be done before that goal is reached (Lee et al. 2021; Su et al. 2022).

While the differences between mental illnesses are undeniable, the commonality between mental illnesses is striking. This has even led to the theory that there is just one common factor "p," the level of which determines the level of psychopathology (Taylor et al. 2023; Caspi and Moffitt 2018; Pettersson et al. 2016). While this may be an oversimplification, it has led to some interesting observations.

According to Caspi and Moffit (2018), one of the leading contenders for p is "the disordered form and content of thought that permeates the extreme of practically every disorder." They go on to list conditions where disordered thought processes are prominent: "affective disorders, anxiety disorders, eating disorders, PTSD, somatoform disorders, dissociative disorders, substance use disorders, and antisocial disorders." By way of explanation, affective disorders include depression and its polar opposite: mania. Somatoform disorders include anxiety, depression, and phobias that manifest themselves through physical symptoms or illness and are commonly referred to as "psychosomatic." Dissociative disorders describe those who have episodes of amnesia, experience self or surroundings as unreal, alternating personalities, etc.

With repeated examinations, it is found that at least 85% of people have a diagnosable mental illness by accepted medical standards at some time in their lives.

Caspi and Moffit suggest that if there is a single p factor, then there ought to be a single treatment. As one possibility, they suggest the numerous forms of cognitive behavioral therapies (CBTs) that are used to treat "eating disorders, anxiety disorders, depression, personality disorders, substance abuse, PTSD, aggression, and psychoses." To us, CBTs make eminent sense as they attempt to educate the mind to improved thoughts and habits where possible.

While mental illness has important consequences for society, one may ask how important it is for us who consider ourselves normal. One answer to this question comes from the study of large numbers of people over time. With repeated examinations, it is found that at least 85% of people have a diagnosable mental illness by accepted medical standards at some time in their lives (Caspi et al. 2020; Schaefer et al. 2017). We say "at least" because the longest period of observation was forty-two years in the Dunedin Study, not a full lifetime (Caspi et al. 2020). Though a large majority of people can be expected to experience mental illness at some point in their lives, in most cases, the illness is limited in severity and can be expected to resolve over time, just as a broken bone heals over time (Schaefer et al. 2017). A minority (about 17%) of the Dunedin Study cohort never received a diagnosis of mental illness during the study. The investigators classified these individuals as experiencing "enduring mental health" and compared them with the majority group participants who were only diagnosed with a mental illness one or two times during the study.

Several factors distinguished enduring mental health (EMH). Those in the EMH group tended to have few relatives with mental illness and not have experienced the loss of a parent or abuse as a child. They also had "fewer emotional difficulties, less social isolation, and superior self-control" (Schaefer et al. 2017). The authors suggest their findings deserve further research. We believe they offer an approach to mental illness prevention and suggest the following as reasonable goals in raising children:

- Teach children they are loved and valued by kindness and discipline.
- Teach children to be friendly.
- Teach children self-control.

Even if these goals should prove insufficient to guarantee mental health, we believe they will contribute to a child's mental health and will in no way prove harmful. It has recently become recognized that mental illness can be prevented to a degree. The appropriate age to begin such efforts is early childhood. A report by the National Research Council and Institute of Medicine (2009) reviews a number of methods that have been put forward to deal with the big three of anxiety, depression, and substance abuse. Most of these methods are forms of cognitive behavioral therapy (CBT) or variations thereon and frequently delivered in a school setting. Many have shown benefits in preventing a fourth or more of cases, but much more research is needed to solidify these results (2009).

While prevention in the young is of undoubted importance, studies examining psychopathology throughout life indicate that the most common illnesses are depression, anxiety, and substance abuse. These often have onset in adults (Kessler et al. 2005; Pettersson et al. 2016; Schaefer et al. 2017). For those who desire to avoid substance use, education is the key. Of particular interest in this regard are two websites maintained by the US Government: https://1ref.us/byb10 is a website for parents, educators, and caregivers; https://1ref.us/byb11 is for anyone and includes true stories contributed by those who have suffered addiction. There seems to be little research on the prevention of anxiety (Krijnen-de Bruin et al. 2022). However, treatments that succeed for depression are often successful for anxiety. It seems to be a reasonable assumption that methods that prevent depression can also prevent anxiety. We will therefore consider depression in more detail.

Depression is the leading cause of disability worldwide (Heissel et al. 2023; Munoz et al. 2012). Many different modalities have been suggested to treat or prevent depression. Generally, more is known about treatment than about prevention, but as a rule, what can treat can also prevent. Antidepressant medication has been a staple of the field for many years. However, a recent analysis of many studies comparing typical medications for depression with placebos reveals that medication is just marginally better than placebo treatment is (Cipriani et al. 2018). If ten people are treated with medication, five will improve, but four of those will improve because of the placebo effect (McCormack and Korownvk 2018).

It has been argued that even this small effect may not be real due to bias and lack of effective blinding in the studies (Kirsch 2019; Moncrieff 2018). Many downsides to taking the medication include "increased risk of relapse, suicidality, gastrointestinal and intracranial bleeding, deep vein thrombosis, pulmonary embolism, diabetes, stroke, epilepsy, and death from all causes" (Kirsch 2019; Almohammed 2022; Bansal 2022; Bielefeldt 2016; Maslej et al. 2017). Because many other treatments are as effective as is the medication in reducing symptoms (e.g., "psychotherapy, physical exercise, acupuncture, omega-3, homeopathy, tai chi, qigong, and yoga" [Kirsch 2019]), medication seems to be a poor choice (Kirsch 2019; Moncrieff 2018). However, if you are on medication, work with your doctor to find an alternative; do not quit on your own, as this could rekindle depressive symptoms.

Because of medication's downside for depression, other methods of treatment have been tried. As already mentioned, many have been found to be equally as effective as medication is without the negative consequences (Kirsch 2019; Khan et al. 2012). Because all these methods are said to be as effective as medication is, but not more effective, it is likely that all of them are acting largely by a placebo effect (Khan et al. 2012). The main requirement for improvement seems to be to enter some kind of therapy. Both diet (Masana et al. 2018; Perez-Cornago et al. 2017) and exercise (Mammen and Faulkner 2013; Singh et al. 2023) are effective against depression, but the benefit beyond placebo may be the general effect that a healthier body makes for a healthier mind (NRCIM 2009, p. 211). As a treatment, the effectiveness of exercise seems to wane over time, which is consistent with a placebo effect (Singh et al. 2023).

Beyond lifestyle factors, there is psychotherapy, of which the most evidence-based approach is CBT. CBT is an umbrella term for approaches that seek to modify counterproductive behaviors and restructure unreasonable and hurtful thinking patterns. The basic approach has been successful for many conditions, including depression, where it is found to equal antidepressant medication in the short term and exceed medication in the long term. CBT roughly cuts relapse rates of depression in half (Kirsch 2019)—likewise with the risk of attempted suicide (Bielefeldt et al. 2016; Gotzsche and Gotzsche 2017). Furthermore, the benefits of CBT as preventative extend over at least five-to-six years (Munoz et al. 2012). However, many people will never enter therapy for various reasons. Self-help resources are available.

For the prevention of depression, bibliotherapy (a form of CBT) can be recommended (Khan et al. 2012; Gualano et al. 2017; Smith et al. 1997; Stice et al. 2010). Two self-help books used for bibliotherapy are *Feeling Good: The New Mood Therapy* by David Burns and *Control Your Depression* by Peter Lewinsohn et al. One reads one of these books and puts into practice its instructions. There are also internet and computerized programs for anxiety and depression that have shown promise as therapy and would be reasonable options for prevention (Newby et al. 2016). For more information on this, we suggest contacting a qualified therapist.

Where needed, CBT is highly recommended as a health-promoting preventative measure. It has the advantage of what we would term a "rational therapy." One is taught to replace aberrant thinking, which depresses the mood with thoughts that are more positive. We believe this is supported by a large GWAS study that provides evidence that more years of education are a prevention of depression. In the same study, a higher IQ did not prevent depression (Wray et al. 2018). Apparently, education provides a certain mental discipline that leads to improved modes of thought. An important question is, To what extent can people learn improved thinking?

Ellen White suffered from depression more than once in her earlier years yet learned to deal with it: "I am sometimes greatly perplexed to know what to do, but I will not be depressed. I am determined to bring all the sunshine into my life that I possibly can" (1977, p. 492). How this was accomplished is explained by other statements. She naturally approached the issue from a spiritual perspective:

Gird up the loins of your mind, says the apostle; then control your thoughts, not allowing them to have full scope. The thoughts may be guarded and controlled by your own determined efforts. Think right thoughts, and you will perform right actions. (*The Adventist Home*, p. 54)

Those who do not feel that it is a religious duty to discipline the mind to dwell upon cheerful subjects will usually be found at one of two extremes: they will be elated by a continual round of exciting amusements, indulging in frivolous conversation, laughing, and joking; or they will be depressed, having great trials and mental conflicts, which they think but few have ever experienced or can understand. (*Mind, Character, and Personality*, vol. 2, p. 487)

If they would train their minds to dwell upon themes which have nothing to do with self, they might yet be useful....

Despondent feelings are frequently the result of too much leisure. The hands and mind should be occupied in useful labor, lightening the burdens of others; and those who are thus employed will benefit themselves also....

The mind should be drawn away from self; its powers should be exercised in devising means to make others happier and better. (*Reflecting Christ*, p. 161)

Controlling the mind is also supported scripturally (see Phil. 4:8; 2 Cor. 10:5). If Christians are more successful in controlling their thoughts, it would be because their faith provides greater motivation.

White also made statements regarding the prevalence of mental illness:

Sickness of the mind prevails everywhere. Nine tenths of the diseases from which men suffer have their foundation here. (*Counsels on Health*, p. 324)

A great deal of the sickness which afflicts humanity has its origin in the mind and can only be cured by restoring the mind to health. There are very many more than we imagine who are sick mentally. Heart sickness makes many dyspeptics, for mental trouble has a paralyzing influence upon the digestive organs. (*Testimonies for the Church*, vol. 3, p. 184)

Nothing is so fruitful a cause of disease as depression, gloominess, and sadness. (*Mind, Character, and Personality*, vol. 2, p. 482)

In closing, we would like to remind ourselves that genetic factors play a significant role in mental illness. People are not created equal physically or mentally. Not everyone with a mental illness is able to help oneself. People with depression may be too depressed to make any effort on their own behalf. Some are afflicted with a form of severe depression that does not respond to standard treatments. Fortunately, new approaches are being developed that have helped such people. One of these is Transcranial Magnetic Stimulation (TMS) (Hutton et al. 2023; Levkovitz et al. 2015). TMS appears to be essentially without serious side effects or adverse health consequences (Levkovitz et al. 2015). If you or a loved one suffers from severe depression and have not found relief, this is an option worth exploring with your physician.

CHAPTER 11

Getting Rest

As one of Job's famous friends said, "For affliction does not come from the dust, nor does trouble spring from the ground; yet man is born to trouble, as the sparks fly upward" (Job 5:6, 7). Some are born with defective bodies or minds; others develop diabetes, asthma, or cancer as children; one can struggle with peer acceptance, bullying, lack of parental care or discipline, or conversely, outright abuse; poverty may be the family's lot; then comes the challenge of graduating from school and finding stable, satisfying employment and raising a family for those fortunate enough to find a spouse. Finally, one will face old age with inevitable deteriorating health and possibly serious financial challenges. And behind all this is the incessant drumbeat of the news media making sure we are aware of the latest mass shooting, storm, flood, fire, or earthquake and the looming catastrophe of another pandemic, global warming, or nuclear war. It does not matter how normal you are. All these things are sources of distress and make it difficult to rest.

Behind all this is the incessant drumbeat of the news media making sure we are aware of the latest catastrophe or war. All these things are sources of distress and make it difficult to rest.

Any distressing thing that happens to us is known technically as a "stressor." Stressors stress the body, and the body responds. Acutely, the mind may respond with anger or fear, and the body will respond with a shot of adrenaline. The result is known as the "fight or flight" reaction. The heart speeds up, blood pressure rises, breathing deepens, muscles tense, blood becomes more able to clot, and the immune system is prepared to resist any invasion of foreign substance. At the same time, digestion is halted, and the adrenal glands secrete cortisol, which begins to shut down inflammatory and repair processes, preparing the body to focus all resources on the perceived threat.

Once the danger is past, all these processes return rather quickly to normal (Salleh 2008). If such reactions are infrequent or mild, they are consistent with good health. We routinely face mild stressors such as bad traffic, defending a viewpoint, giving a speech, or chairing a committee. The body is built for such things, and the experience may be exhilarating. In such cases, the stress has the nickname "eustress." It is when major stressors are encountered chronically that health is likely to be impacted negatively.

Studies of people who have experienced major chronic life stressors, either as children or in adulthood, reveal an increased risk for many illnesses, including depression, digestive and gastrointestinal problems, hypertension, diabetes, cardiovascular disease, autoimmune diseases, loss of bone minerals, immunosuppression, asthma, upper respiratory infections (URIs), and poorer wound healing (Salleh 2008; Cohen et al. 2012; Morey et al. 2015), as well as dementia (James et al. 2023). While the consequences of chronic stress are well documented, how disease is produced is less understood.

Under chronic stress, epinephrine (adrenalin) is not continually secreted. Cortisol, however, can remain elevated for some time but eventually returns to a normal level. As a result, one cannot detect the presence of chronic stress in many cases by observing cortisol levels. Instead, evidence indicates that chronic stress is correlated with decreased sensitivity to cortisol (Cohen et al. 2012). Since one of cortisol's functions is to dampen the immune reaction and resulting inflammation, in chronic stress, inflammation tends to operate at a higher level and with less control. This can presumably be the basis for an increased prevalence of many chronic diseases (*Ibid.*).

The sympathetic nervous system consisting of nerve ganglia located along the spinal column and sending nerve branches to all parts of the body, including the adrenal glands, is responsible for reacting to stress. Fortunately, the body also has a parasympathetic nervous system consisting of nerves that run: with the third cranial nerves to the eyes; with the seventh and ninth cranial nerves to the lacrimal and salivary glands and the mucous membranes of the mouth and upper airway; with the tenth (i.e., vagus) nerves to the heart, lungs, and gastrointestinal tract; and from the sacral portion of the spinal cord to the distal part of the colon, rectum, kidneys, bladder, gonads, and external sex organs.

The parasympathetic system opposes the sympathetic system and is responsible for bringing the body back to its normal resting state after experiencing an acute stressor. Both systems are part of the autonomic nervous system, which means generally, they do what they do without conscious control on one's part. Where the sympathetic system raises the heart rate and blood pressure, the parasympathetic system lowers both. The result tends to be a healthy balance when things are working properly.

Because of the prevalence of chronic stress with its negative health consequences, it is important to look for ways either to reduce the stress or counter it by activating the parasympathetic nervous system. One can approach the problem of stress in many ways that have proven to be somewhat beneficial. The direct approach of raising the activity level of the parasympathetic system can be accomplished by progressive relaxation (Merakou et al. 2019), deep abdominal breathing exercises (Toussaint et al. 2021), increasing heartrate variability with breathing through biofeedback (Goessl et al. 2017; Taghizadeh 2019), or exercise (Fontana et al. 2022; Jacquart 2019).

Heartrate variability with breathing is a complicated function of many factors (Malik 1996), but sympathetic and parasympathetic tone are major factors. One can learn to increase the parasympathetic tone relative to the sympathetic tone through biofeedback and thereby calm the nerves. Exercise is effective because during active exercise, the sympathetic nervous system activates and is more ready to rest after activity. Furthermore, exercising muscles send signals for the vegetative and digestive functions supported by the parasympathetic system, causing it to be activated, especially post-exercise. Beyond what I have called the "direct approach," there are numerous distractive approaches that help one to ignore the sources of stress to an extent. Among these are music therapy (de Witte 2022; Erbay Dalli et al. 2022), aromatherapy (Son 2019), art therapy (Reynolds and Sova 2022), and various forms of meditation (Schlechta Portella et al. 2021).

We view meditation as distractive because the common way it is practiced is known as "mindfulness meditation." In a careful, academically-acceptable definition, mindfulness meditation consists of two guiding principles:

1. "The self-regulation of attention so that it is maintained on immediate experience, thereby allowing for increased recognition of mental events in the present moment.…

2. "Adopting a particular orientation toward one's experiences in the present moment, an orientation that is characterized by curiosity, openness, and acceptance" (Bishop et al. 2004).

Mindfulness is a practice to be learned. The practitioner develops the skill of keeping the mind focused on breathing or some other aspect of the present moment and learns to observe and acknowledge intruding thoughts, feelings, or sensations but not pursue them or criticize them (Fontana et al. 2022; Jacquart 2019). The goal is to always come back to the object of focus in the present moment. We do not doubt that mindfulness meditation relieves stress to an extent. An important question is whether it is better than competing methods are. This is an issue that has not received much study. However, one study examining physical activity, mindfulness meditation, and heartrate variability training with biofeedback found the three methods equally effective in reducing stress (van der Zwan et al. 2015). More studies are needed before definitive conclusions can be drawn.

Our concern with mindfulness meditation is the directive to allow thoughts to take place unchallenged. As a Christian, we believe it is important to simply outlaw some thoughts from the mind. Most Christians, we believe, will understand this reservation. One could also be concerned about the Buddhist roots of mindfulness meditation, but the Western interpretation thereof leaves out any reference to Buddhism (Bishop et al. 2004). Consequently, we believe mindfulness meditation can be acceptable to the Christian when modified to exclude acceptance of thoughts outlawed by the biblical standard. We personally do not practice mindfulness meditation and prefer physical exercise and deep breathing exercises as good ways of producing relaxation under stressful conditions.

In some cases, one can remove a chronic stressor from one's experience. In this case, the adage "an ounce of prevention is worth a pound of cure" applies. One such situation is the matter of overwork. Global competition has given rise to a feverish desire to outperform one's competitors. In Japanese, there are words for some of the consequences: "*Karoshi* (sudden death caused by cardiovascular or cerebrovascular disease due to overwork) and *karojisatsu* (suicide due to overwork)" (Bannai and Tamakoshi 2014). Overwork as long hours has been noted as a source of depression, anxiety, cardiovascular disease, cancer, diabetes, and substance abuse (Bannai and Tamakoshi 2014; Atroszko et al. 2020). Those with obsessive-compulsive disorder (OCD) have been identified as high risk for overwork due to rigid perfectionism or obsession with productivity. It is theorized that those affected have difficulty recognizing overwork as a problem (Atroszko et al. 2020).

Unfortunately, people who work excessive hours do not necessarily benefit from doing so. Results of the Whitehall II study, conducted for five-and-a-half years, showed that middle-aged British civil servants who worked over fifty-five hours per week experienced a decline in their vocabulary and reasoning skills when compared with those who worked forty hours per week at most (Virtanen et al. 2009).

Regarding productivity, studies of munitions workers in Britain and the USA during World War II showed the effect of long working hours on productivity. In one large British factory, workers were assigned to work seventy-four hours per week but were only able to attain sixty-six. When the assignment was cut to sixty-four hours per week, workers succeeded in working fifty-four, but production did not decrease. Subsequently, workers were assigned to work fifty-four hours per week and succeeded in working forty-eight, but to the amazement of all, production increased by 13% for women and 19% for men.

In an American factory, work hours were increased from ten to twelve hours per day, and production fell by 6.5 %. Based on these and other observations, some general conclusions were drawn: 1) Every reduction in the working day leads to a decrease in accidents, spoiled work, sickness, and absence; 2) the reduction of working hours from twelve to ten leads to an increase in hourly and daily output; and 3) the reduction of working hours from ten to eight leads to a further increase in hourly and daily output, except in operations whose speed depends mainly on the speed of machines (Sayers 1942).

The war also taught a lesson regarding the ability of humans to work consistently seven days a week. Winston Churchill stated in the House of Commons on July 29, 1941:

> First of all, if we are to win this war—and I feel solidly convinced that we shall—it will be largely by staying power. For that purpose you must have reasonable minimum holidays for the masses of the workers. There must, as my hon. Friend himself urged in his speech, be one day in seven of rest as a general rule, and there must be, subject to coping with bottle-necks and with emergencies which know no law, a few breaks and where possible one week's holiday in the year. ("Hansard Committee Debate")

Surely, these lessons should not be lost on us.

Ellen White had important counsel regarding the management of stress and the conditions of labor. One area of concern pertained to deep breathing and its ability to relax the nervous system and promote health:

Next in importance to right position are respiration and vocal culture. The one who sits and stands erect is more likely than others to breathe properly. But the teacher should impress upon his pupils the importance of deep breathing. Show how the healthy action of the respiratory organs, assisting the circulation of the blood, invigorates the whole system, excites the appetite, promotes digestion, and induces sound, sweet sleep, thus not only refreshing the body, but soothing and tranquilizing the mind. And while the importance of deep breathing is shown, the practice should be insisted upon. Let exercises be given which will promote this, and see that the habit becomes established. (*Education*, p. 198)

The physician should teach the patient how to breathe deeply, and this in many cases will be found to be a means of healing. (*Manuscript Releases*, vol. 3, p. 309)

White clarified what she meant by deep breathing in another statement regarding patient education: "Encourage them to breathe the fresh air. Teach them to breathe deeply, and in breathing and speaking to exercise the abdominal muscles. This is an education that will be invaluable to them" (1905, p. 264).

She saw physical exercise as an important aspect of caring for the mind and keeping the activity of the nervous system in a healthy balance:

The time spent in physical exercise is not lost.... A proportionate exercise of all the organs and faculties of the body is essential to the best work of each. When the brain is constantly taxed while the other organs of the living machinery are inactive, there is a loss of strength, physical and mental. The physical system is robbed of its healthful tone, the mind loses its freshness and vigor, and a morbid excitability is the result....

Those who are engaged in study should have relaxation. The mind must not be constantly confined to close thought, for the delicate mental machinery becomes worn. The body as well as the mind must have exercise. (*The Adventist Hope*, p. 494)

White saw special benefit in exercise obtained through useful labor:

There are many amusements that excite the mind, but depression is sure to follow. Other modes of recreation are innocent and healthful;

but useful labor that affords physical exercise will often have a more beneficial influence upon the mind, while at the same time it will strengthen the muscles, improve the circulation, and prove a powerful agent in the recovery of health. (*Counsels on Health*, p. 627)

Long hours of work without rest were considered particularly harmful:

> Those who make great exertions to accomplish just so much work in a given time, and continue to labor when their judgment tells them they should rest, are never gainers. They are living on borrowed capital. They are expending the vital force which they will need at a future time. And when the energy they have so recklessly used is demanded, they fail for want of it.… Their time of need has come, but their physical resources are exhausted. Everyone who violates the laws of health must sometime be a sufferer to a greater or less degree.…
>
> It is not our duty to place ourselves where we shall be overworked. Some may at times be placed where this is necessary, but it should be the exception, not the rule.… If we honor the Lord by acting our part, He will on His part preserve our health.… By practicing temperance in eating, in drinking, in dressing, in labor, and in all things, we can do for ourselves what no physician can for us. (White, *My Life Today*, p. 142)

> Let no one labor to the point of exhaustion, thereby disqualifying himself for future effort. Do not try to crowd into one day the work of two. At the end, those who work carefully and wisely will be found to have accomplished as much as those who so expend their physical and mental strength that they have no deposit from which to draw in time of need.…
>
> God is merciful, full of compassion, reasonable in His requirements. He does not ask us to pursue a course of action that will result in the loss of physical health or the enfeebling of the mental powers. He would not have us work under a pressure and strain until exhaustion follows, with prostration of the nerves. (White, *Gospel Workers*, p. 244)

Ellen White was also an advocate of rest beyond limiting the hours worked in a day. As a Seventh-day Adventist, she naturally advocated keeping the biblical weekly Sabbath.

> Heaven's work never ceases, and men should never rest from doing good. The Sabbath is not intended to be a period of useless inactivity.

The law forbids secular labor on the rest day of the Lord; the toil that gains a livelihood must cease; no labor for worldly pleasure or profit is lawful upon that day; but as God ceased His labor of creating, and rested upon the Sabbath and blessed it, so man is to leave the occupations of his daily life, and devote those sacred hours to healthful rest, to worship, and to holy deeds. The work of Christ in healing the sick was in perfect accord with the law. It honored the Sabbath. (*The Desire of Ages*, p. 207)

She also recommended that sedentary workers, when possible, take an occasional day to relax:

Let the whole day be given to recreation. Exercise in the open air, for those whose employment has been within doors and sedentary, will be beneficial to health. All who can should feel it a duty to pursue this course. Nothing will be lost, but much gained. They can return to their occupations with new life and new courage to engage in their labor with zeal, and they are better prepared to resist disease. (*Counsels on Health*, p. 196)

In summary, we recommend an approach to stress control that consists of four parts: First, limit the time worked each workday to eight hours. This will limit exhaustion and allow time for other needful duties and still provide time for seven or eight hours of sleep each night. Second, if work is sedentary, spend at least thirty minutes a day in moderate-to-vigorous exercise. This will reduce the effects of stress on the body. Also learn to breath slowly and deeply using the abdominal muscles in breathing. When feeling stressed, take ten slow, deep breaths to experience the relaxation it brings. Third, be sure one day a week is spent on activities other than work. For this purpose, we recommend keeping the biblical Saturday Sabbath free from labor. This will give the nerves used in daily labor a chance to rest and rejuvenate before beginning the weekly work grind again. Finally, we have found that several weeks a year away from work and responsibilities is great for renewing the energies of body and mind.

CHAPTER 12

My Quest for Health

Why would you or anyone else want to hear about my life? Perhaps because I believe aspects of my quest for health might be instructive. As true with many Adventists, I grew up a vegetarian. Our family was poor, with four kids to feed. My dad never wanted to work for anyone but himself. Working for himself consisted largely in buying and selling used equipment and junk, which never seemed to net much profit. When necessary, he harvested fruit or worked in other farm labor to provide needed income. We usually had sufficient food, but most of it was prepared at home from basic ingredients. We usually had a cow for milk. At times, we even had some chickens that provided eggs to supplement our diet.

We never had money to see a doctor or dentist on a regular basis, but we did receive the recommended vaccines such as DPT, smallpox, and polio. My mother had a severe bout with sciatica at one point, and my father was afflicted with pneumonia at another time. (A doctor friend came to our house and gave him a shot of penicillin, which got him back on his feet.) We children all had chickenpox, measles, mumps, and German measles at a young age. I do not recall anyone being treated for strep throat. For the most part, our family remained healthy when I was a child.

Why would you or anyone else want to hear about my life? Perhaps because I believe aspects of my quest for health might be instructive.

It was while I was in high school that Mom took a job running a health food store. The wheelchair-bound owner needed help to take some time off and start a second health food store in another location some distance away. We began to experience different kinds of foods, such as royal jelly, wheat germ, flax seed, brewer's yeast, and seaweed, with purported health benefits. Mom had always baked our bread herself, but now we experienced different kinds of bread with seeds, nuts, etc. Many books and magazines with varied claims regarding health were also sold.

Because the owner was an Adventist, books on health by Ellen G. White were for sale. Because Dad was interested in health, Mom often brought home applicable literature. At one point, Dad read someone's book about the herb comfrey and began growing it, grinding up the leaves with other herbs, and drinking the result. It is now known that comfrey contains carcinogenic pyrrolizidine alkaloids that can cause liver failure if ingested in sufficient quantity (Stickel and Seitz 2000). I don't recall that he became ill from ingesting comfrey, but it did not do wonders for him either. Eventually, he read the writings of someone who claimed that the best health was achieved by eating only uncooked food. From that point on, he would rarely eat anything that had been cooked. Any effort to reason with him on the issue was time wasted.

In his younger days, Dad had been a supporter of White's counsels on health, but at this point, they seemed to carry no weight with him. He was unmoved by statements such as this:

> No one should adopt an impoverished diet. Many are debilitated from disease, and need nourishing, well-cooked food. Health reformers, above all others, should be careful to avoid extremes. The body must have sufficient nourishment. The God who gives His beloved sleep has furnished them also suitable food to sustain the physical system in a healthy condition. (*Counsels on Diet and Foods*, p. 91)

By putting forth his ideas Dad alienated his fellow church members and, deciding they had treated him harshly, he ceased to attend our local church. All of this led me to look more into what I could learn about health. I read White's writings on health and even had my mother obtain a book on metabolism from the public library so I could learn how many calories a person needed to eat to remain healthy. I was quite impressed with what I was learning and tried to put it into practice.

When I attended college, I continued practicing my health habits, except I believe I would have benefitted from getting seven or eight hours of sleep each night instead of trying to exist on six. The first three years, I had a job involving physical labor to help pay my expenses, which helped me. In my senior year, I had a sedentary job and am convinced that I would have been healthier had I gotten more physical exercise. I did well academically, but one can always improve. More exercise and sleep would have made for better health and very likely led to improved performance. As it was, I did well enough in college to obtain a university fellowship to study mathematics at the University of California, Davis.

My wife and I lived in student housing near the campus where we could ride bicycles a couple miles to and from classes. This provided needed exercise. I believe my sleep habits improved. I also did well in graduate school and credit much of that to my health habits. I wrote a 133-page thesis entitled "On Non-absolute Integration in Topological Spaces" and finished my degree in a little over two years. When I returned to my alma mater to teach mathematics, I tried to convince my students of the benefits of a healthy lifestyle. I believe some benefited.

I taught mathematics for five years and then decided to enroll in medical school. Even though I was interested in research, I felt the field of medicine was a place where it would be easier to make a practical difference in people's lives. I had entertained some ideas regarding my health that were quickly corrected when I entered medical school. One of these ideas revolved around low blood sugar. I had read a book that claimed many of the world's problems could be blamed on low blood sugar. I became convinced I suffered from the problem. When I mentioned it to one of the doctors in the clinic for students, I was invited to volunteer for a blood glucose test the next time I felt my sugar was low. I did so, and the test showed my sugar was very normal. I learned that low blood sugar is quite rare unless one is diabetic and on medication that can lower the levels. Other causes are rare indeed.

Another concern was low thyroid function. I had been told by a physician that I needed thyroid hormone and was taking it regularly, but that turned out to be incorrect also. My thyroid gland was working normally. Mom, based on her reading of literature at the health food store, had started using hydrochloric acid tablets, which were supposed to help digestion. I thought I needed them too. In pharmacology class, I learned that the amount of acid they contained was miniscule compared with the amount the stomach produced. I did not need those pills either.

These changes did not have much effect on my health, but they did change my perception of my health. Again, I tried to exist on six hours of sleep a night during my basic science years. I am convinced it would have been smarter to aim for more sleep at the expense of study time. During my clinical years, sleep was often at a premium. There was no solution except to sleep whenever one had a chance. I went on to do an internship and residency in internal medicine. Sleep deprivation was a way of life during those years. I can remember many morning reports when my brain felt numb; it was a challenge to sound rational much less articulate in describing the patients admitted during the previous night.

After my residency, it was my privilege to be awarded a fellowship in the Mathematical Research Branch of the NIADDK (back when the institute lumped arthritis, digestive diseases, and kidney diseases together) at the National Institutes of Health in Bethesda, Maryland. However, I had one year between when my residency ended and the fellowship began, so I worked full-time as an ER doctor for the Kaiser Foundation Hospital in Sacramento, California. After that, I spent three very enjoyable years doing research. During this time, I had the privilege of working with Dr. David Lipman, who came to the Math Research Branch six months after I did. He was interested in biological sequence analysis, and together we did some important research, which included co-publishing six papers. During this time, I often worked one night shift per week in an ER to help with finances. We had three sons, and all attended a private church school.

Upon completion of my fellowship, I took a job working the night shift Monday through Friday in an ER near where we lived. This required no investment on my part, and the pay was good, but I found it difficult to obtain the needed sleep. I worked at this job for five years. During this time, my marriage dissolved, so I moved into a cool, quiet basement condo that allowed for refreshing sleep. It was tolerable. Eventually, I was forced to move and rented a third-floor condo that was noisy and had inadequate cooling. It was difficult. If you work the night shift and attempt to sleep during the day, it is important to have the best sleeping conditions possible. The ideal place would be a cave—cool, dark, and quiet.

One day, I received a phone call from my former colleague David Lipman. He remained at NIH and had been appointed the director of a newly established National Center for Biotechnology Information (NCBI), which was tasked by Congress with the job of collecting and making available to the public the growing biological sequence data that were just beginning to be produced at many research institutions domestically and globally. I was excited to join this new group in 1989 in its second year, when there were about a dozen employees. I believe there are now about 400 employees, which is a testament to how the data collection and the complexity of caring for it have grown over the years.

Shortly after joining NCBI, I married Bonnie Burns. She has been a faithful partner and a great help. Not long after we were married, she mentioned getting a migraine headache every Monday morning. I pointed out to her that one thing that can improve migraines is keeping regular hours for meals and sleep. I offered to fix breakfast every day if she would get up and join me for breakfast. She took me up on the offer and no longer suffered migraines from sleeping in on weekends. I still fix breakfast thirty-three years later.

My youngest son came to live with us at one point while in college. I noticed he did not follow regular hours for eating and sleeping. He also seemed to be having some trouble with his schoolwork. I offered him $1,000 if, for one academic semester, he would follow regular times for eating and sleeping, including getting to bed in time to get a reasonable amount of sleep. He agreed, and things began to improve for him academically. (At the same time, he wanted to buy a motorcycle. I refused to help him buy a motorcycle but offered to pay half the cost for a used car. I had seen the carnage that can befall young riders in my work in emergency medicine.)

Over the years since our marriage, Bonnie and I have been quite heavily involved in volunteer work at our church. I was head elder for nineteen years, am still an elder, and have regularly taught a Bible study class for years. Bonnie teaches a women's group, oversees fellowship meals, takes turns preparing PowerPoint slides for services, and often plays the violin with the praise team. Together we have offered several seminar series on living a healthy lifestyle for the public as well as our church. In these ventures, Bonnie has concentrated her efforts on seeing that healthy food is served at the event while I have given a doctor's perspective on healthy life habits. Such efforts are always interesting for us, and there is a certain satisfaction that comes from doing something that benefits others. Research has shown that volunteering confers health benefits (Piliavin and Siegl 2007; Yeung et al. 2017), especially if the work is undertaken with the purpose of benefitting others.

For most of my life, I would rate my health as excellent. I have been on no regular medication and have rarely used any medicine. I don't take vitamins regularly (I believe pregnant women can benefit from taking vitamins, but the evidence suggests most people do not [Chen et al 2019]). Ellen White counseled, "In grains, fruits, vegetables, and nuts are to be found all the food elements that we need" (1938, p. 92). As far as herbs are concerned, I have found a cup of warm peppermint tea enjoyable at times because it can sooth the stomach and intestines.

Bonnie has suffered from osteoarthritis of the knee. She tried steroid shots with some benefit, but it proved to be short-lived. Her dermatologist suggested trying turmeric, and she has been taking 1,000 milligrams per day for over a year and has felt much relief. Another kind of treatment we have both found helpful is something we simply describe as hot-and-cold treatments. For this we use a Thermophore pad. It produces moist heat when plugged into an outlet. Beyond that, one needs a good ice bag. My approach is to fill the ice bag with about fifteen cubes and then add cold water until the bag is about half-full. Then a treatment is given by applying the Thermophore hot enough to be uncomfortable for three minutes. This is then followed by applying the ice bag to the same area for three minutes. This is repeated three times to make a full treatment.

The heat brings blood to the area, and the cold drives the blood away. In this way, toxins from an inflamed or infected site can be washed away while fresh immune cells are brought in. This can greatly help clear up an infection or heal a wound. It can provide relief for the common cold or sore throat. I don't know if it shortens a cold but it can certainly make one feel better. I am convinced I once cured pneumonia using such treatments on my chest. Another time, I tried the same technique without success.

In the past, I suffered from a frozen shoulder and used hot-and-cold treatments as described here to successfully treat the inflammation and pain. Once the pain and tenderness had resolved, I did stretching exercises until the shoulder was functional again. I am not recommending this as an ideal approach but simply giving my experience. My version of hot-and-cold treatments is adapted from the book *Manual of Hydrotherapy and Massage* (Moor et al. 1964, pp. 51, 52). Because medical problems are not always what they seem, it is important that you see a medical professional and follow his or her directions for your care. If you are interested in hot-and-cold treatments, you should discuss your interest with the doctor.

One thing with which I have suffered is irritable bowel syndrome of the constipating variety. For this I drink about three-and-a-half cups of water at just below 120°F when I first rise in the morning. One must avoid a burn, but this temperature is well within the safe range for normal people, and it is essential that the water be quite warm to have a laxative effect. Then I will drink another large glass of warm water an hour before a meal later in the day. I find this generally helpful.

Eating prunes is also helpful if needed. As I have gotten older, I have found it beneficial to take MiraLAX or an equivalent with my water in the morning. Everyone is different, so what works for me is not guaranteed to work for others, but I suspect it will benefit some. I came to drink water in the morning based on an Ellen White statement: "I should bathe frequently, and drink freely of pure, soft water.... Water can be used in many ways to relieve suffering. Drafts of clear, hot water taken before eating (half quart, more or less), will never do any harm, but will rather be productive of good" (1938, p. 419).

Even though the water from the public water system is considered pure, we have distilled the water we use for drinking or cooking for many years. We consider this an added protection against the possibility of some unsuspected pollutant like PCBs showing up in the future. Some people with irritable bowel syndrome find it helpful to avoid certain foods that are a source of gas and/or abdominal discomfort. Such foods are generally termed "FODMAPs" (fermentable oligosaccharides, disaccharides, monosaccharides and polyols); one can easily find a list on the internet. I have not personally found such a list helpful, but I do find Beano helpful when eating beans.

Probably sometime between 2005 and 2010, I was sitting in my office when I suddenly experienced a pressure in my chest that rapidly increased until it was severe and vise-like. As a physician, I knew this was a typical symptom of a heart attack. However, I found it hard to believe I could really be having a heart attack. I have always had a normal electrocardiogram and have never had a high LDL cholesterol level. After all, I was a vegetarian, regularly exercised, had regular hours for eating and sleeping, with at least seven hours of sleep a night. I knew esophageal spasms could cause pain simulating a heart attack. However, the discomfort did not let up, and I began

Physicians are known for not taking very good care of themselves. I am afraid I fit the mold. I am forced to admit it is very likely I was experiencing the early stage of a heart attack.

to concede that I should ask someone to call 911, but I was feeling weak. At that point, I simply fell back in my chair and whispered, "Lord save me!" Within less than two minutes, the symptoms I was feeling completely disappeared. At that point, I was extremely relieved yet unable to entertain the thought that this was a heart-related event.

I simply assumed it was something else and said nothing to anyone. I did not want to pursue something I did not believe could be serious. Physicians are known for not taking very good care of themselves. I am afraid I fit the mold. I should have at least pursued the issue with some tests. Given what I would later learn about my coronary arteries, I am forced to admit it is very likely I was experiencing the early stage of a heart attack, which would have killed me had the merciful God whom I serve not intervened and given me a reprieve. God does promise there will be health benefits to those who serve Him.

> There He made a statute and an ordinance for them, and there He tested them, and said, "If you diligently heed the voice of the Lord your God and do what is right in His sight, give ear to His commandments and keep all His statutes, I will put none of the diseases on you which I have brought on the Egyptians. For I *am* the Lord who heals you." (Exodus 15:25, 26)

Though I was trying to serve the Lord as well as live in a healthy manner, all the years of working night shifts were sufficient reason to suspect heart disease. Shift work is a known risk factor. Regarding healing, Ellen White had this to say: "It is labor lost to teach people to look to God as a healer of their infirmities, unless they are taught also to lay aside unhealthful practices.… They must live in harmony with the law of God, both natural and spiritual" (1905, pp. 227, 228). I can claim no perfection, but I have found the Lord to be merciful.

I officially retired as a government employee in November 2015. After retirement, I continued to work part-time as a contractor with the same colleagues with whom I had worked at NCBI and contribute to research projects important to the goal of providing services to the public. I continued because I loved the work but, at age seventy-three, felt the need to slow the pace. I continued my efforts to live a healthy lifestyle. It was about 2018 when I began to feel my legs were getting weak. I seemed to have some trouble with walking in a steady manner.

At around that time, I was researching exercise as a way of improving longevity and came upon the studies described in chapter 7 of this book. Improving maximal exercise capacity could increase longevity and was some insurance against serious disease. I found REHIT an appealing approach to improve maximal exercise capacity. I decided to put it into practice on our elliptical exercise machine: three-minute warm up, twenty-second all-out sprint, three-minute active recovery, twenty-second all-out sprint, and three-minute cool down. I repeated this roughly ten-minute routine Mondays, Wednesdays, and Fridays, lifted weights on Tuesdays, Thursdays, and Saturdays, and just did mild exercise on the elliptical on Sundays. After a few weeks, I found my legs were much stronger and my gait was steady.

On December 1, 2021, I awoke at 5 a.m. as usual and, shortly thereafter, descended to the basement and started my REHIT routine. However, I found myself very weak and completely unable to do the sprints. Finally, I got off the elliptical exercise machine, sat down, and took my pulse. My pulse rate was 73 but very irregular. I realized my heart was in atrial fibrillation. I experienced no chest pain, but that does not rule out a serious event such as a heart attack. I immediately went upstairs and asked Bonnie to drive me to the emergency room of the local Adventist hospital, which is close to our home.

When we arrived, my cardiogram was normal, and tests did not show any evidence of heart damage. I was seen by a cardiologist who decided to admit me because of my age and perform some additional tests. This was the first night I had ever spent in a hospital as a patient. The next day, a 2D echo and nuclear stress test were performed and were normal. I was discharged with a wearable heart monitor, which I wore for two weeks. This also showed nothing abnormal. During the next couple months, I experienced two more brief episodes of atrial fibrillation. My cardiologist diagnosed paroxysmal atrial fibrillation and placed me on the blood thinner Rivaroxaban for stroke prevention. He also suggested I get a CT Calcium Score of my coronary arteries. This was positive at a moderate level of 226, with all but 11 coming from my left main and left anterior descending arteries. He placed me on a statin.

A few months later, I noticed a discomfort in my throat when walking up a hill, which had not previously been a problem. I thought I recognized this feeling as something I had experienced doing my REHIT routine. I had assumed it was from the cold morning air. Walking at midday, the air was not cold. The problem got progressively worse. It was then clear to me that I was suffering from exertional angina. I toyed with the idea of trying a dietary approach (no added fats, nuts, or animal products). I decided it was most important to get testing done to see the extent of the problem and what the treatment options were.

My cardiologist put me on the schedule for an angiogram. The angiogram showed 90% blockage of my left main coronary artery. The doctors judged my case too critical to allow me to leave the hospital, and I had triple vessel bypass surgery three days later on September 16, 2022. During the surgery, my atrial appendage was clipped and an ablation was done on the left atrium with the goal to prevent further problems with atrial fibrillation. My recovery was uneventful.

About three months after my surgery, Bonnie and I traveled to South Carolina to spend the winter. We have a small condo near Huntington Beach State Park. Shortly after arriving, I began to have trouble sleeping. I was having trouble breathing when lying in bed, and my ankles were showing some swelling. I finally went to a local emergency room and received the diagnosis of early heart failure, which I expected. A 2D echocardiogram of my heart did not show any segmental wall motion abnormalities, which suggested the grafts remained functional. I was given a prescription for Lasix at a low dosage and offered follow-up with a local cardiologist.

One of our favorite activities when we visit South Carolina is walking on the beach at Huntington Beach State Park (we look for fossil sharks' teeth and enjoy seeing the many different creatures that inhabit the beach and surrounding woodlands). We usually walk a couple miles on the beach each day, but I soon found I could not walk that far without getting severely out of breath. The distance shortened to one-and-a-half miles, one mile, half a mile, and then some days, I was too weak to walk at all. We cut short our vacation, packed our bags, and headed home. I would normally share the driving with Bonnie, but I was not able to drive.

I followed up with my cardiologist, and a 2D echocardiogram was performed. A stress test was planned, but when my cardiologist looked at the echo, he saw severe pulmonary hypertension. He canceled the stress test and placed me again on a blood thinner, thinking I was experiencing pulmonary emboli (blood clots forming in my legs and moving to my lungs and blocking the flow of blood). He ordered a CT scan of my lungs with contrast. This was done, and there was no evidence of blood clots. He then thought I might have Dressler's syndrome and placed me on medication usually used to treat gout. This medication made me so sick that it was finally discontinued at my request.

Regardless, on a Sunday morning in late March, I was so weak that I asked Bonnie to take me to the emergency room. Tests soon showed that both my blood sodium and potassium levels were seriously low and both lungs were bathed in fluid, making it difficult for me to breathe. I was admitted to the hospital where the blood levels of sodium and potassium could be addressed. A needle was inserted next to my right lung and 1.8 liters of fluid were removed and sent for tests. There was no sign of infection, but neither was there any clue as to why the excess fluid was accumulating. I was discharged home on Lasix.

Within a week, I was back in the emergency room. My potassium was normal, but my sodium was even lower than it was before. My right lung was surrounded by both air and fluid, making breathing difficult. A chest tube was placed in the right side of my chest, and I was admitted to the hospital. During the first two hours after the chest tube was placed, two-and-a-half liters of fluid were removed, as well as air. I felt great relief.

However, the fluid continued to drain from the right side of my chest with no sign of stopping.

After six days, the chest tube was removed and replaced with a small semi-permanent catheter that could be used to drain fluid even at home if needed. The mystery of why the fluid was accumulating remained until one of the cardiologists who specialized in the use of CT angiograms ordered this test on my ninth day in the hospital. The test showed I had significant pulmonary vein stenosis in at least three of my four pulmonary veins. This is a rare complication occurring in about 1% of those who have had an ablation, as I had had at the time of my surgery.

The University of Maryland Medical Center (UMMC) in Baltimore runs a pulmonary hypertension treatment center, and a physician at the center had accepted me as a patient, but no bed had become available. I remained in the Adventist hospital as a patient for another eight days. While waiting for a bed, additional tests were done to confirm the diagnosis, including another CT scan to examine the fine structure of the lungs and a simultaneous left and right heart catheterization. A bed was still not available at UMMC. Many prayers were ascending for me during this time.

Finally, it was decided that I would be discharged home where we would wait for word from the Washington Hospital Center in Washington, DC, to put me on their schedule for the procedure I needed. The specialist, Dr. Michael Slack, who could treat my problem, had privileges there as well as at UMMC. Going home would be necessary because the Washington Hospital Center does not accept transfers from hospitals in Maryland. I was still feeling quite weak, with the fluid draining from my chest at over a liter a day.

Bonnie was fearful of how we could manage. If we could not manage, we were to drive to the Washington Hospital Center and go to the emergency room for treatment. While I was receiving a last bolus of fluid and albumin before discharge, the charge nurse suddenly appeared with the news that a bed had opened up at UMMC. We were overjoyed and thanked God for answered prayer. I was transferred late that evening.

At UMMC, the cardiology team saw me at once, but Dr. Slack was on vacation and would return in a week. He was, however, consulted in regard to my care. It was agreed that I should have another simultaneous right and left heart catheterization to rule out constrictive pericarditis as another possible cause of my condition. This was done, and while the test was not completely normal, it was decided that the abnormalities were not clinically meaningful. I finally received treatment from Dr. Slack on May 2. He was able to place five stents in my four pulmonary veins. Only the right upper vein was completely blocked, but he was able to insert a wire, open it up, and place two stents.

As I was waking up from the anesthesia, I noticed my right hand felt numb with a tingling sensation. I asked the nurse about it. She immediately showed interest. I then noticed my left arm felt like it was lying across my chest, but when I felt it with my right hand, it felt like a sausage and was at my left side! I could not feel it or move it. The cardiology fellow on duty as well as a radiology fellow rushed me to get a CT angiogram of my head and neck to rule out a stroke. The scan proved normal. When Dr. Slack heard of the problems with my arms, he said he had seen this before and described them as due to brachial plexus injuries.

During the procedure, it was necessary to move both of my arms above my head and keep them there for over three hours. Because both of my shoulders have been frozen in the past, they do not move easily above my head. Fortunately, both arms improved quite rapidly. The right one is now normal while the left is near normal. Once the stents were placed, the drainage from the chest catheter diminished greatly but not sufficiently enough to have it removed. I remained in the hospital a few days while follow-up care for the catheter was arranged. I was finally discharged home after thirty-three days in the two hospitals.

How do I think about this recent illness, and what does it say about living a healthy lifestyle? Pulmonary vein stenosis is a known but rare complication of the ablation procedure, which was done during my triple vessel bypass. I am clearly what one might call unlucky. However, there is no guarantee that one will avoid such a complication. Solomon wisely said, "I returned and saw under the sun that—The race *is* not to the swift, nor the battle to the strong, nor bread to the wise, nor riches to men of understanding, nor favor to men of skill; but time and chance happen to them all" (Eccles. 9:11). Not everyone who suffers serious health complications has lived an unhealthy lifestyle.

Ellen White made an interesting statement in relation to this issue: "A failure to care for the living machinery is an insult to the Creator. There are divinely appointed rules which if observed will keep human beings from disease and premature death" (1938, p. 16). One must ask what premature death is. Is White saying if we really follow a healthy lifestyle, we will *never* get any disease and simply die of "old age," which is presumably not a disease? Or is she saying if we follow a healthy lifestyle, we will not succumb to a disease prematurely. I lean toward the latter.

Solomon suggested we all can expect to come to a time in our lives when life is unrewarding. "Remember now your Creator in the days of your youth, before the difficult days come, and the years draw near when you say, 'I have no pleasure in them'" (Eccles. 12:1). Arguably, death at that point is not premature.

White herself was a careful health reformer for many years, but she died of a stroke at age eighty-seven. If we take the biblical statement as a guide, we have a possible answer: "The days of our lives *are* seventy years; and if by reason of strength *they are* eighty years, yet their boast *is* only labor and sorrow; for it is soon cut off, and we fly away" (Ps. 90:10). Perhaps even if we live a healthy lifestyle and are fortunate enough to avoid health problems brought on by our genes or uncontrollable environmental factors, we can only reasonably expect seventy or eighty good years. Anything beyond that should be considered a gift.

Most of us will die of a disease at some point. That means most of us will be sick at some point. Christ said, "Those who are well have no need of a physician, but those who are sick" (Luke 5:31). While healing could be the result of a miracle, we believe it is more likely to come by correcting unhealthy life habits or, in some other way, removing the cause of disease. The apostle Paul, in listing the gifts of the Spirit, gives "gifts of healings" and "the working of miracles" each a place (1 Cor. 12:9, 10).

According to Ellen White, "There were physicians in Christ's day and in the days of the apostles. Luke is called the beloved physician. He trusted in the Lord to make him skillful in the application of remedies" (1958, p. 286). She did not hesitate to recommend treatment to the sick.

> If you are sick, you should call in a physician. (*Manuscript Releases*, vol. 12, p. 98)

> If there is need of a surgical operation, and the physician is willing to undertake the case, it is not a denial of faith to have the operation performed. After the patient has committed his will to the will of God, let him trust, drawing nigh to the Great Physician, the Mighty Healer, and giving himself up in perfect trust. The Lord will honor his faith in the very manner He sees is for His own name's glory. "Thou wilt keep him in perfect peace, whose mind is stayed on Thee: because he trusteth in Thee. Trust ye in the Lord for ever: for in the Lord Jehovah is everlasting strength." (*Selected Messages*, book 2, p. 284)

I think it is safe to conclude that even when living a healthy lifestyle, most of us will need the services of a physician at some point.

There is the question of what exactly is the healthiest lifestyle. To this question, we do not believe there is a single answer. As White expressed it:

There is a wide difference in constitutions and temperaments, and the demands of the system differ greatly in different persons. What would be food for one, might be poison for another; so precise rules cannot be laid down to fit every case. I cannot eat beans, for they are poison to me; but for me to say that for this reason no one must eat them would be simply ridiculous. I cannot eat a spoonful of milk gravy, or milk toast, without suffering in consequence; but other members of my family can eat these things, and realize no such effect; therefore I take that which suits my stomach best, and they do the same. We have no words, no contention; all moves along harmoniously in my large family, for I do not attempt to dictate what they shall or shall not eat. (*Counsels on Diet and Foods*, p. 494)

> *There is the question of what exactly is the healthiest lifestyle. To this question, we do not believe there is a single answer.*

Foods that are palatable and wholesome to one person may be distasteful, and even harmful, to another. Some cannot use milk, while others thrive on it. Some persons cannot digest peas and beans; others find them wholesome. For some the coarser grain preparations are good food, while others cannot use them. (p. 198)

The benefits of a healthy lifestyle should speak for themselves.

Those who understand the laws of health, and who are governed by principle, will shun the extremes, both of indulgence and of restrictions. Their diet is chosen, not for the mere gratification of appetite, but for the upbuilding of the body. They seek to preserve every power in the best condition for the highest service to God and man. The appetite is under the control of reason and conscience, and they are rewarded with health of body and mind. While they do not urge their views offensively upon others, their example is a testimony in favor of right principles. These persons have a wide influence for good. (p. 198).

My understanding of a healthy diet is that it should satisfy four principles:

1. It should be composed of natural ingredients.

2. Ingredients should be combined in a simple manner.

3. The resulting food should be appetizing.

4. It should impart strength to those who partake.

I believe these points are supported by science as well as the counsels of Ellen White. In our time, some advocate for no animal products or even go a step further and add the requirement of no nuts or oils in the diet. If this kind of diet works for you, I have nothing to say. However, in our experience, we have found it quite difficult to prepare appetizing food without eggs, dairy products, nuts, or added oils. I strongly suspect the benefit of going without eggs, dairy products, nuts, and oils is primarily weight lost and has relatively little to do with the composition of the diet beyond that. As far as I know, this is a question calling for research. In any case, it is important to remember the goal of health reform is improved health and strength. White expressed it well:

> Because it is wrong to eat merely to gratify perverted taste, it does not follow that we should be indifferent in regard to our food. It is a matter of the highest importance. No one should adopt an impoverished diet. Many are debilitated from disease, and need nourishing, well-cooked food. Health reformers, above all others, should be careful to avoid extremes. The body must have sufficient nourishment....
>
> Let it ever be kept before the mind that the great object of hygienic reform is to secure the highest possible development of mind and soul and body. (*Counsels on Diet and Foods*, pp. 199, 464)

Alternatively, Solomon expressed it this way: "Blessed *are you*, O land, when your king *is* the son of nobles, and your princes feast at the proper time— for strength and not for drunkenness!" (Eccles. 10:17).

I am now 81 years old, and based on my experience, I believe I have gained much from the counsels of Ellen White. As the years have gone by, I have seen them more and more confirmed by science, as I have tried to explain in these pages. I am convinced that God gave her a gift of knowledge, not only because I see the scientific evidence, but also because of her humble attitude regarding this gift. She never presented herself as some great authority.

I have had great light from the Lord upon the subject of health reform. I did not seek this light; I did not study to obtain it; it was given to me by the Lord to give to others. I present these matters before the people, dwelling upon general principles, and sometimes, if questions are asked me at the table to which I have been invited, I answer according to the truth. But I have never made a raid upon any one in regard to the table or its contents. I would not consider such a course at all courteous or proper. (*Counsels on Diet and Foods*, p. 493)

Here is an example we should all seek to emulate.

CHAPTER 13

Another Look at Science

Up until this point, we have looked at science as it relates to health and seen how it has given us guidance to a healthier lifestyle. Much of what we have learned was anticipated in the writings of Ellen White in the nineteenth and early twentieth centuries, and we have tried to show these correlations where possible. This history largely explains how Seventh-day Adventists came into possession of principles for healthy living that have stood the test of time. With that said, science has a broader scope than health alone.

An important question is, What are the limits of science? Some claim science makes religion irrelevant. White was aware of this claim and wrote insightfully on the subject. Here we will look at what sound reasoning and research has shown regarding the limitations of science and again attempt to correlate this with insights from her writings. In the end, we believe there are health implications. A healthy religion makes for a healthy mind. "For God has not given us a spirit of fear, but of power and of love and of a sound mind" (2 Tim. 1:7).

As the definition of "science," the *Oxford English Dictionary* states it is "the systematic study of the structure and behavior of the physical and natural world through observation, experimentation, and the testing of theories against the evidence obtained." *Merriam-Webster* defines science as "knowledge or a system of knowledge covering general truths or the operation of general laws especially as obtained and tested through scientific method." Based on these definitions, we will define scientific knowledge as general truths or laws that make testable and potentially falsifiable predictions about the physical world. As Karl Popper pointed out, theories that make no falsifiable predictions are not scientific theories because they cannot be false (1968).

As defined, scientific knowledge has a broad sweep. The very fabric of rationality and the essence of our comfort in the world is the ability to predict. From a very young age, we possess something we call "knowledge" that allows us to predict. We know the sun comes up every morning and sets about twelve hours later. Given this knowledge, we can predict some of what we see happening. We know if we place an object at a certain spot in a room, it will very likely be there later. Common-sense knowledge like this makes us feel comfortable in this place where we live.

However, predictability runs much deeper. It is a rigorous test of scientific knowledge and useful knowledge in general. Newton's laws of motion have been of great practical use as they allow us to predict the motions of physical bodies. They have, in a sense, been superseded by Einstein's relativistic theories because the latter make more accurate predictions under certain extreme conditions. The current cutting edge of physical knowledge is in particle physics. Based on the Standard Model of particle physics, physicists predicted the existence of the Higgs Boson in 1964. In 2012, CERN's Large Hadron Collider confirmed its existence, giving a strong confirmation to the theory (Jakobs and Seez). We are not aware of any practical consequences of this knowledge other than the satisfaction of human curiosity—the desire to know.

Chemistry is largely about the consequences of mixing certain substances. This knowledge is used to our advantage in creating many useful products. Likewise, knowledge of the predictable consequence of applying certain chemicals to living organisms is the foundation of much medical practice as well as the science of agriculture. Journalists are valued because their knowledge allows them to predictably write articles that people will take the time to read. A similar statement can be made regarding many other professions and the value of their knowledge. Based on these observations, we may conclude that predictability is very fundamental to our existence.

We see scientific knowledge as a bright star in the galaxy of human endeavor. It promises good for humanity. However, we are convinced there are times when science makes claims that will not stand up to rigorous examination. In 1999, the US National Academy of Sciences put forth the following statement: "For those who are studying the origin of life, the question is no longer whether life could have originated by chemical processes involving nonbiological components. The question instead has become which of many pathways might have been followed to produce the first cells."

A more honest statement comes from a University of Chicago commentary on recent efforts to understand the origins of life on our planet: "The origin of life on Earth stands as one of the great mysteries of science. Various answers have been proposed, all of which remain unverified" (Koppes 2022).

There are reasons to question any scenario that claims to provide proof that life came about by strictly natural means. An important one is our ignorance about what constitutes life. There is not one living cell type for which we can say we understand in detail how it functions. As David Berlinski says, "No one has the faintest idea whether the immense gap between what is living and what is not may be crossed by any conceivable means" (Berlinski 2009).

A second point of contention is the claim that Darwin's theory of evolution by natural selection is responsible for the development of the known life forms from a simple common ancestor. Presumably, no informed person would controvert the claim that natural selection is a force in nature. The controverted issue pertains to the limits of what natural selection can accomplish in modifying organisms. All living organisms from humans on down are built largely of protein molecules with the addition of some RNA molecules. Both protein molecules and RNA molecules are specified by the genes of the organism. The genes in total make up the genome, which is somewhat equivalent to a large instruction book. Such an instruction book can contain a large amount of information.

The likelihood of a random process producing this simple protein molecule is about the same as the chance of tossing a coin and getting heads 300 times in a row.

Hubert Yockey (1977) has shown that even for a quite simple protein, cytochrome c, the amount of information is about 300 bits. Bits can be thought of as coin tosses, and a random process can be expected to produce a cytochrome c molecule with about the same probability as tossing a fair coin 300 times and obtaining heads at every toss. You have probably heard of lifting oneself up by one's bootstraps. How well would it work if you and a colleague tried to lift each other up by the bootstraps at the same time. Not likely!

Well, suppose we are given a hospitable, natural environment and just two simple organisms that are to compete. Each is essentially providing the environment for the other. Then what is the chance that by random mutation and natural selection, they will develop new, sophisticated information in their genomes (instruction books)? From where would such sophisticated information come? Can they really lift each other up by the bootstraps, so to speak? It is by no means a given, even with unlimited time.

The biochemist Michael Behe has pointed out that for Darwinian theory to be a credible account of the development of life, it must account for the development of sophisticated biological mechanisms at the molecular level. He terms such mechanisms "examples of irreducible complexity," which he defines: "By irreducibly complex I mean a single system composed of several well-matched, interacting parts that contribute to the basic function, wherein the removal of any one of the parts causes the system to effectively cease functioning" (2019).

As examples, he suggests the protein gyrase, the bacterial flagellum, and the vertebrate blood-clotting system. Recent advances in technology now allow the rapid sequencing of DNA and proteins and have opened the way for studies to examine how natural selection functions in real biological systems. The results were unexpected. "The amazing but in retrospect unsurprising fact established by the diligent work of many investigators in laboratory evolution over decades is that the great majority of even beneficial positively selected mutations damage an organism's genetic information—either degrading or outright destroying functional coded elements" (Behe 2019).

This is unsurprising because there are far more ways for a single mutation to damage or destroy a gene product or control sequence than there are ways for such a mutation to improve it. Damage somewhere in the genome is often sufficient to provide a selective advantage to an organism in some environment. This is observed to be true, not only in the laboratory but also in studies of organisms in their natural environments. On the other hand, no one has yet succeeded in demonstrating the evolution of a sophisticated new molecular function involving multiple genetic changes (Behe 2019).

Eugene Koonin is a careful molecular biologist with a long history of studying the genomes of diverse organisms. He has concluded that the Darwinian picture of life is incorrect: "Major transitions in biological evolution show the same pattern of sudden emergence of diverse forms at a new level of complexity. The relationships between major groups within an emergent new class of biological entities are hard to decipher and do not seem to fit the tree pattern that, following Darwin's original proposal, remains the dominant description of biological evolution" (2007).

Koonin points to RNA and protein molecules as the most fundamental. Of these, there are many different sizes and shapes with different functions, but there is no evidence that one type morphed into another type. Likewise, there are different classes of viruses, but it is not clear that one or a few types of these viruses are the ancestors of the others. And so on, up the proposed hierarchy of organisms, until one reaches the multicellular organisms and the different animal phyla. Researchers cannot agree on trees or even which came first.

"In each of these pivotal nexuses in life's history, the principal 'types' seem to appear rapidly and fully equipped with the signature features of the respective new level of biological organization. No intermediate 'grades' or intermediate forms between different types are detectable" (Koonin 2007). This picture of what is actually seen in nature seems consistent with what Behe sees, though Behe and Koonin are at opposite ends of the spectrum regarding origins. In response, Koonin proposes a series of what he calls "Biological Big Bangs" in which somehow, new biological information (molecules) is generated rapidly by natural processes, but the mechanism(s) for this remain highly speculative (2007).

> When consideration is given to man's opportunities for research; how brief his life; how limited his sphere of action; how restricted his vision; how frequent and how great the errors in his conclusions, especially as concerns the events thought to antedate Bible history; how often the supposed deductions of science are revised or cast aside; with what readiness the assumed period of the earth's development is from time to time increased or diminished by millions of years; and how the theories advanced by different scientists conflict with one another,—considering all this, shall we, for the privilege of tracing our descent from germs and mollusks and apes, consent to cast away that statement of Holy Writ, so grand in its simplicity, "God created man in His own image, in the image of God created He him"? Genesis 1:27. Shall we reject that genealogical record,—prouder than any treasured in the courts of kings,—"which was the son of Adam, which was the son of God"? Luke 3:38. (White, *Education*, p. 130)

After describing the fact that religion proposes answers to "the great and aching questions of life, death, love, and meaning," David Berlinski asserts, "I do not know whether any of this is true. I am certain that the scientific community does not know that it is false" (2009). For me, the apostle Paul's statement rings true:

> For since the creation of the world His invisible *attributes* are clearly seen, being understood by the things that are made, *even* His eternal

power and Godhead, so that they are without excuse, because, although they knew God, they did not glorify *Him* as God, nor were thankful, but became futile in their thoughts, and their foolish hearts were darkened. (Romans 1:20, 21)

Human knowledge of both material and spiritual things is partial and imperfect; therefore many are unable to harmonize their views of science with Scripture statements. Many accept mere theories and speculations as scientific facts, and they think that God's word is to be tested by the teachings of "science falsely so called." 1 Timothy 6:20. The Creator and His works are beyond their comprehension; and because they cannot explain these by natural laws, Bible history is regarded as unreliable. Those who doubt the reliability of the records of the Old and New Testaments too often go a step further and doubt the existence of God and attribute infinite power to nature. (White, *The Great Controversy*, p. 522)

Which is better, the faith that attributes all power to nature and believes that sometime in the future, someone will explain how life began and how it has proliferated on this earth by some natural process, or the faith that believes in a Creator God who created all things, animate and inanimate?

A third point of scientific contention is how earth's geologic record should be interpreted. Up until about 200 years ago, geologists were generally convinced that the geologic record held significant evidence of what could be termed "catastrophic" events. As Victor Baker has explained, this changed when Charles Lyell's treatise came on the scene. Lyell was impressed with the theories of James Hutton and John Playfair, who appear to have been strongly influenced by Isaac Newton's approach to physics. In his *Principia*, Newton had advocated for principles of simplicity and economy in assumptions. Lyell expressed his understanding applied to geology:

My work ... will endeavour to establish the principle of reasoning in the science; and all my geology will come in as illustration of my views on those principles, and as evidence strengthening the system necessarily arising out of the admission of such principles ... (the principles being) that no causes whatever have ... ever acted, but those now acting; and that they never acted with different degrees of energy from that which they now exert ..." (Charles Lyell, "Letter to Roderick Murchison, Esq. (15 Jan. 1829)," in *Life, Letters and Journals of Sir Charles Lyell, Bart*, vol. 1, p. 234)

This is the uniformitarian basis for the science of geology, which is strongly held to this day. It firmly closes the door against a worldwide flood as an explanation for the earth's geological formations. Lyell felt there was an unwarranted, religiously motivated bias towards catastrophism in the geology of his day and took pains to guard against it in his *Principles of Geology*.

Victor Baker is himself a staunch proponent of catastrophism and describes his approach: "Catastrophism in the Earth sciences is rooted in the view that Earth signifies its causative processes via landforms, structures and rock. Processes of types, rates and magnitudes not presently in evidence may well be signified this way" (1998). Through his careful fieldwork and that of others, the Channeled Scabland of east-central Washington state, as well as features of the Martian landscape, have become accepted as consequences of cataclysmic flooding. This was only possible when it was recognized that the relevant geological features could only be the consequences of the "high-energy physics" of mega-flooding (2009).

The same reasoning can be applied on an even broader scale. Ariel Roth observes, "The incredibly widespread flat sedimentary formations and the layers within them, the lack of evidence for long ages at the flat gaps between sedimentary layers, and the abundance of material from oceans on the continents are powerful worldwide factors that very much favor the Flood model of the Bible" (Geoscience Research Institute, https://1ref.us/byb12, July 8, 2014). Here, flat gaps are areas where one would have expected three geological formations, A, B, and C, with A appearing on top of B, which should in turn be on top of C. However, B is missing, and A appears smoothly on top of C, with virtually no erosion at the interface. On the standard geological time scale, the missing formation(s) B can represent a few million to as much as 200 million years (Roth 2009).

There are reasons why current geological formations may provide insufficient information to determine history. Many natural processes lead to greater disorder over time. This is predicted by the second law of thermodynamics for a closed system (https://1ref.us/byb13 [last modified February 6, 2024]). A closed system is one in which energy is not flowing in or out of the system. For our purposes, it seems reasonable to consider the earth and its atmosphere essentially a closed system because the amount of radiation flowing in and out seems unlikely to have had any appreciable effect to decrease the disorder of the earth-atmosphere system during the formation of its geological features.

For example, incident sunlight would not be expected to appreciably decrease the havoc wrought by earthquakes, hurricanes, tornadoes, floods, or volcanic activity. If entropy is increasing, then information is being lost; it is not possible to recover this information, and we have no way to say what exactly the state was before entropy increased (i.e., we have no way to recover history). This argument is clearly most relevant when the processes at work have been catastrophic. There is also the argument based on chaos theory, which tells us that complicated non-linear physical systems are very likely governed by chaotic dynamics (https://1ref.us/byb14 [last modified February 16, 2024]).

We cannot construct proof of the biblical flood. By the same token, those who believe earth's features required billions of years cannot prove their case.

If this is true, prediction of future states becomes impossible beyond some time limit. This is why weather prediction is only accurate out to about one week (and sometimes significantly less), but if you cannot predict the weather more than a week ahead, then neither can you start with the current weather and use the equations for weather prediction to reason backwards and say what the weather was more than a week ago. You may know what the weather was more than a week ago, but that could only be true if you (or someone else) recorded it. The same is very likely true of the earth's geological history.

Ellen White, in commenting on geological history, made the following statement:

> But apart from Bible history, geology can prove nothing. Those who reason so confidently upon its discoveries have no adequate conception of the size of men, animals, and trees before the Flood, or of the great changes which then took place. Relics found in the earth do give evidence of conditions differing in many respects from the present, but the time when these conditions existed can be learned only from the Inspired Record. (*Patriarchs and Prophets*, p. 112)

We may think that if the biblical flood described in Genesis actually happened fewer than 5,000 years ago, we should be able to prove it by looking at the rocks and sediments we see currently covering the earth. This statement by White suggests we cannot construct such a proof. By the same token, those who believe earth's geological features, including the fossil-bearing rocks, required millions or billions of years to accumulate will also not be able to prove such is the case.

I have presented these arguments concerning the origins of life on earth, the diversity of life, and the geological features of the earth to convince you, the reader, that solid science does not rule out the existence of God and His claimed creatorship and agency in our world. I would also like to convince you that the Bible gives evidence you can examine for yourself of a Power that our human science cannot comprehend.

God even invites you to examine His claims. "Remember the former things of old, for I *am* God, and *there is* no other; *I am* God, and *there is* none like Me, declaring the end from the beginning, and from ancient times *things* that are not *yet* done" (Isaiah 46:9, 10).

As humans, we have a very limited ability to predict the future. We can predict the weather with some accuracy for a few days, but the accuracy decreases rapidly with the increased time period involved. To predict tomorrow's news headlines is quite beyond our abilities. God has made some long-range predictions, however. Let us examine several.

First, in Daniel 2, God lays out the future for Nebuchadnezzar, Daniel, and all those who might read his book. Besides the kingdoms of Babylon (605–539 BC) and Medo-Persia (539–331 BC), the prediction is that two more kingdoms would rule the world. First would be Greece (331–168 BC), who would wrest power from Medo-Persia. In turn Greece, would fall before the iron kingdom of Rome. Rome ruled the world from 168 BC until AD 476. Daniel 2 tells us this fourth kingdom would eventually be divided, with some parts strong and some parts weak.

We understand the divisions to be the so-called barbarian tribes that filled the power vacuum when Rome fell. Daniel goes on to say, "As you saw iron mixed with ceramic clay, they will mingle with the seed of men; but they will not adhere to one another, just as iron does not mix with clay" (2:43). This refers to the long history of intermarriage between the royal houses of Europe (Benzell and Cooke 2021) and says in spite of this effort to unite the countries involved, it would not succeed, but they would remain as a mixture of strong and weak countries as we see today. The next thing Daniel saw is the end of history, when God sets up His kingdom.

Another fascinating prophecy is given in Isaiah 44–45, where the prophet names Cyrus as one whom God would raise up to be king, free His people from captivity, and command the rebuilding of Jerusalem and the restoration of its temple. So that Cyrus would know God is God and there is none like Him, God even gives details of how Cyrus would be able to conquer Babylon:

Thus says the Lord to His anointed, to Cyrus, whose right hand I have held—to subdue nations before him and loose the armor of kings, to open before him the double doors, so that the gates will not be shut: "I will go before you and make the crooked places straight; I will break in pieces the gates of bronze and cut the bars of iron. I will give you the treasures of darkness and hidden riches of secret places, that you may know that I, the Lord, who call *you* by your name, *am* the God of Israel. For Jacob My servant's sake, and Israel My elect, I have even called you by your name; I have named you, though you have not known Me. I *am* the Lord, and *there* is no other; *There is* no God besides Me. I will gird you, though you have not known Me, that they may know from the rising of the sun to its setting that *there is* none besides Me. I *am* the Lord, and *there is* no other; I form the light and create darkness, I make peace and create calamity; I, the Lord, do all these *things*." (Isaiah 45:1–7)

Amazingly, this prophecy was given over 100 years before Cyrus came on the scene! The Greek historian Herodotus stated that on the night when Cyrus captured Babylon, a festival was taking place, and the city gates along the Euphrates were not closed as people were to be allowed to cross the river at will (Livius, https://1ref.us/1at, [last modified July 14, 2020]). Daniel 5 gives the account of the fall of Babylon and indicates there was a feast taking place and the capture of the city was a surprise to the Babylonian king, Belshazzar. This and the Isaiah passage above, which states "the gates will not be shut," lend some credence to Herodotus' statement.

After Cyrus captured Babylon, he made a decree to let the captive Israelites go free, that they might return to Jerusalem and rebuild God's temple. Interestingly, in the decree he states that "all the kingdoms of the earth has the LORD God of heaven given me. And He has commanded me to build Him a house at Jerusalem which is in Judah" (2 Chronicles 36:23, Ezra 1:2). Evidently, Cyrus was sufficiently impressed by Isaiah's prophecy that he acknowledged the God of heaven as the origin of his success. That is no small admission for a heathen king. We should be equally impressed. This is like someone in Abraham Lincoln's day giving the name of the person who will be US president in the year 2024.

Another amazing prophecy was written by King David. This prophecy gives certain details pertaining to the crucifixion of Christ. It begins with the words "My God, My God, why have You forsaken Me?" (Ps. 22:1), spoken by Jesus on the cross. A few verses on are the words "All those who see Me ridicule Me; they shoot out the lip, they shake the head, *saying*, He trusted in the LORD, let Him rescue Him; let Him deliver Him, since He delights in Him!" (verses 7, 8).

These verses are very reminiscent of the words recorded at the crucifixion scene:

> Likewise the chief priests also, mocking with the scribes and elders, said, "He saved others; Himself He cannot save. If He is the King of Israel, let Him now come down from the cross, and we will believe Him. He trusted in God; let Him deliver Him now if He will have Him; for He said, 'I am the Son of God.'" Even the robbers who were crucified with Him reviled Him with the same thing. (Matthew 27:41–44)

"They pierced My hands and My feet" (Ps. 22:16). This clearly refers to the nails driven through Christ's hands and feet at His crucifixion. As far as we know, crucifixion was a form of punishment invented by the Persians circa 500 BC. This is about 500 years after Psalm 22 was written. Again, "They divide My garments among them, and for My clothing they cast lots" (verse 18; see Matt. 27:35). Who but God could inspire the writing of these words 1,000 years before the events took place.

Finally, consider this prophecy: "Then I said to them, 'If it is agreeable to you, give *me* my wages; and if not, refrain.' So they weighed out for my wages thirty *pieces* of silver. And the LORD said to me, 'Throw it to the potter'—that princely price they set on me. So I took the thirty *pieces* of silver and threw them into the house of the Lord for the potter" (Zech. 11:12, 13). The events described here are an enigma. No explanation is given of why the money is to be thrown to the potter or why this is done in the house of the Lord.

Nevertheless, events took place in connection with the betrayal of Christ by Judas that make plain the purpose of this passage in Zechariah. It is a prophecy of Judas' behavior in the betrayal and the events following it (see Matt. 27:3–10; Acts 1:16–20). Judas betrayed Christ for thirty pieces of silver, expecting Him to assert His power and become king, but seeing that Christ allowed Himself to be condemned, Judas was filled with remorse and, going to the priests, stated that he had sinned in betraying innocent blood. Their hearts were untouched, and they brushed him off. He then cast the money down in the temple, went out, and hanged himself.

The priests then consulted regarding what to do with this money that was the price of blood and decided to use it to buy a potter's field they had proposed as a place where they can bury dead strangers. The purchase was made, and the field became known as the Field of Blood. Thus, Christ's enemies became the unwitting means of fulfilling the prophecy of Zechariah, and the mysterious connection between thirty pieces of silver, the Lord's house, and a potter becomes clear.

All of this reveals the divine power that can predict minute details of events hundreds of years before they take place. That divine power is the power that claims authorship of Scripture. It is a power so far beyond our human science that it should claim our awe, reverence, and worship. What knowledge is this that allows One to unerringly make such predictions? "For *as* the heavens are higher than the earth, so are My ways higher than your ways, and My thoughts than your thoughts" (Isa. 55:9).

Dear reader, the Bible predicts that the end of the world is coming: "And in the days of these kings the God of heaven will set up a kingdom which shall never be destroyed; and the kingdom shall not be left to other people; it shall break in pieces and consume all these kingdoms, and it shall stand forever" (Dan. 2:44). If we are unprepared, it will come on us unexpectedly: "But the day of the Lord will come as a thief in the night, in which the heavens will pass away with a great noise, and the elements will melt with fervent heat; both the earth and the works that are in it will be burned up" (2 Peter 3:10).

Nevertheless, Jesus has a message of hope for all of us: "Behold, I am coming quickly! Blessed *is* he who keeps the words of the prophecy of this book" (Rev. 22:7). The message of Revelation is designed to prepare people for Christ's return. Seventh-day Adventists believe it is their mission to help anyone who wants to understand the book and prepare for Christ's return. If it is your desire to understand Revelation's message, contact a nearby Seventh-day Adventist church.

CHAPTER 14

A Higher Science

While science seems to make daily gains in new discoveries, it has shown little effectiveness in dealing with the great problems of our time: incessant war, bloodshed, and lawless behavior. These problems are not new, but they are not lessening. There seems to be a serious blight on the human spirit. We may feel superior. How secure are we? Whole societies have turned to bloodthirstiness at the behest of brutish leadership. Might we succumb as well? Most would agree that humanity has a spiritual problem. I understand there are many who believe true spirituality is available from many sources, but I beg you to hear me out.

> *Science seems to make daily gains in new discoveries, it has shown little effectiveness in dealing with the great problems of our time.*

If you had a defective heart valve and were given three weeks to live, where would you go: to a witch doctor, a shaman, or a heart surgeon who could repair your heart? To put it simply, if you have a real problem, you need a real solution. As Christ stated, "Those who are well have no need of a physician, but those who are sick. I did not come to call *the* righteous, but sinners, to repentance" (Mark 2:17). Jesus offers the only credible solution to the sin problem that plagues our world. He offers to take away our guilt and give us a new motivation for living a life patterned after His own. This is all set forth in God's Word: "The Bible is God's great lesson book, His great educator. The foundation of all true science is contained in the Bible. Every branch of knowledge may be found by searching the word of God. And above all else it contains the science of all sciences, the science of salvation. The Bible is the mine of the unsearchable riches of Christ" (White 1900, p. 107).

In the coming moments, we will set forth important elements of the science of salvation.

The Gospel

At the announcement of Christ's birth, the purpose of His coming was given: "And she will bring forth a Son, and you shall call His name JESUS, for He will save His people from their sins" (Matt. 1:21). How this was to be accomplished was set forth in the new covenant:

> But this *is* the covenant that I will make with the house of Israel after those days, says the Lord: I will put My law in their minds, and write it on their hearts; and I will be their God, and they shall be My people. No more shall every man teach his neighbor, and every man his brother, saying, "Know the Lord," for they all shall know Me, from the least of them to the greatest of them, says the Lord. For I will forgive their iniquity, and their sin I will remember no more. (Jeremiah 31:33, 34)

Christ's shed blood put the new covenant into effect, as He made clear at the last supper: "For this is My blood of the new covenant, which is shed for many for the remission of sins" (Matt, 26:28). The new covenant is mentioned again in Hebrews 8, where Christ is presented as ministering its benefits.

Nothing will change until a need for change is recognized. This recognition is the first step toward salvation. When Jesus met the Pharisee Nicodemus at night and told him he needed to be born again, Nicodemus struggled with the idea (see John 3:1–17). In this meeting, Christ laid out conditions for being a part of His kingdom. One must be born of water and the Spirit along with believing in Jesus. Likewise, when Peter preached Christ to the multitude on the day of Pentecost and they were convinced of their sin, the prescription was the same: Repent and be baptized in the name of Jesus for the remission of your sins, and you, too, will receive the baptism of the Spirit (see Acts 2:37, 38). When Paul met Christ on the Damascus road and was convicted of his sins, Christ sent Ananias to minister to him. He was admonished to arise and be baptized to wash away his sins (see 22:16) and receive the Holy Spirit (see 9:17).

From these examples, we see how the two promises of the new covenant are fulfilled. Baptism by water represents the washing away of our sins; they are forgiven and will be remembered no more. Baptism by the Spirit represents the writing of God's law on our heart. "Clearly you are an epistle of Christ, ministered by us, written not with ink but by the Spirit of the living God, not on tablets of stone but on tablets of flesh, *that is*, of the heart" (2 Cor. 3:3). The same thought is expressed in the Old Testament: "I will give you a new heart and put a new spirit within you; I will take the heart of stone out of your flesh and give you a heart of flesh" (Ezek. 36:26). Another way to see the same point is to note that the first fruit of the Spirit is love (see Gal. 5:22) and "love does no harm to a neighbor; therefore love *is* the fulfillment of the law" (Rom. 13:10).

At this point, you may be thinking, 'What about John 3:16?' Does not belief in Jesus guarantee eternal life? The test is whether your belief leads to a love-driven, righteous life (see Rom. 10:10). Can the Holy Spirit turn your faith into love (see Gal. 5:5, 6)? If you believe Jesus loves you personally, the Spirit can turn that into love for Him. "We love Him because He first loved us" (1 John 4:19). Under the control of that love, you will not hesitate to confess Jesus before humanity (see Rom. 10:10). Those who deny Him before humanity fail love's test, and Jesus will not be able to accept them into His kingdom (see Matt. 10:33).

This is an issue for the would-be followers of Christ because those who truly follow Christ witness against the evil in the world and excite the hatred and persecution of the world (see John 15:18–16:4). Peter initially failed this test (see Matthew 26:69–75) but was converted through his experience and restored to his place among the disciples (see John 21:15–19). This issue of loyalty is stated elsewhere by Christ in different verbiage. "If anyone comes to Me and does not hate his father and mother, wife and children, brothers and sisters, yes, and his own life also, he cannot be My disciple. And whoever does not bear his cross and come after Me cannot be My disciple" (Luke 14:26, 27). God has always been a jealous God and unwilling to share His place with other gods (see Exod. 20:5).

It is not sufficient to believe in the historical Christ. The important thing to understand is that believing in Christ means believing His words and putting them into practice. If we forget this, we have misunderstood the Physician's prescription and have no right to expect a cure. Christ said to His hearers:

> But why do you call Me "Lord, Lord," and not do the things which I say? Whoever comes to Me, and hears My sayings and does them, I will show you whom he is like: He is like a man building a house, who dug deep and laid the foundation on the rock. And when the flood arose, the stream beat vehemently against that house, and could not shake

it, for it was founded on the rock. But he who heard and did nothing is like a man who built a house on the earth without a foundation, against which the stream beat vehemently; and immediately it fell. And the ruin of that house was great. (Luke 6:46–49)

Some may protest that this sounds like salvation by works. The apostle Paul confirmed it is not: "For by grace you have been saved through faith, and that not of yourselves; *it is* the gift of God, not of works, lest anyone should boast. For we are His workmanship, created in Christ Jesus for good works, which God prepared beforehand that we should walk in them" (Eph. 2:8–10). The apostle John, speaking of Christ, told us He "loved us and washed us from our sins in His own blood" (Rev. 1:5) and "we love Him because He first loved us" (1 John 4:19). Love leads to efforts to please Christ our Lord. Nevertheless, Christ makes it clear that we are not to think this gives us merit. "So likewise you, when you have done all those things which you are commanded, say, 'We are unprofitable servants. We have done what was our duty to do'" (Luke 17:10). All the power is from Christ through His indwelling Spirit. "For the law of the Spirit of life in Christ Jesus has made me free from the law of sin and death" (Rom. 8:2).

The Relationship

Consider two events that occurred in Christ's day:

There were present at that season some who told Him about the Galileans whose blood Pilate had mingled with their sacrifices. And Jesus answered and said to them, "Do you suppose that these Galileans were worse sinners than all *other* Galileans, because they suffered such things? I tell you, no; but unless you repent you will all likewise perish. Or those eighteen on whom the tower in Siloam fell and killed them, do you think that they were worse sinners than all *other* men who dwelt in Jerusalem? I tell you, no; but unless you repent you will all likewise perish." (Luke 13:1–5)

This is a profound statement by Christ. He is stating that the world has just two classes of people. Those who do not fear God or repent are allowed to receive what life brings. Those who fear God and repent receive only what God allows. While death is the lot of all, "Precious in the sight of the LORD is the death of His saints" (Ps. 116:15). God always has a benevolent purpose in what He allows to happen to His people. For this reason, we are admonished, "In everything give thanks; for this is the will of God in Christ Jesus for you" (1 Thess. 5:18). Even in dying, the righteous experience God's mercy through the blessed hope in a resurrection. Thus, Balaam's inspired statement: "Let me die the death of the righteous, and let my end be like his!" (Num. 23:10).

God has always had a policy of mercy and blessing for those who walk according to His directions. We are told, "And Enoch walked with God; and he *was* not, for God took him" (Gen. 5:24). Likewise, "Noah walked with God" (6:9), and the Lord saved only him and his family in that generation. Many scriptures make this clear:

> For I, the Lord your God, *am* a jealous God, visiting the iniquity of the fathers upon the children to the third and fourth *generations* of those who hate Me, but showing mercy to thousands, to those who love Me and keep My commandments. (Exodus 20:5, 6)

> I command you today to love the Lord your God, to walk in His ways, and to keep His commandments, His statutes, and His judgments, that you may live and multiply; and the LORD your God will bless you in the land which you go to possess. (Deuteronomy 30:16)

> But take careful heed to do the commandment and the law which Moses the servant of the Lord commanded you, to love the Lord your God, to walk in all His ways, to keep His commandments, to hold fast to Him, and to serve Him with all your heart and with all your soul. (Joshua 22:5)

> And I prayed to the LORD my God, and made confession, and said, "O Lord, great and awesome God, who keeps His covenant and mercy with those who love Him, and with those who keep His commandments." (Daniel 9:4)

> And I said: "I pray, LORD God of heaven, O great and awesome God, *You* who keep *Your* covenant and mercy with those who love You and observe Your commandments." (Nehemiah 1:5)

Notice it is always love that leads to the keeping of God's commandments. As Jesus expressed it, love for God is synonymous with keeping God's commandments:

> He who has My commandments and keeps them, it is he who loves Me. And he who loves Me will be loved by My Father, and I will love

him and manifest Myself to him.... If anyone loves Me, he will keep
My word; and My Father will love him, and We will come to him and
make Our home with him. He who does not love Me does not keep
My words; and the word which you hear is not Mine but the Father's
who sent Me. (John 14:21–24)

The same thought is expressed by the apostle John: "For this is the love of
God, that we keep His commandments. And His commandments are not
burdensome" (1 John 5:3).

Christ introduced fascinating symbolism to describe the relationship
between Himself and His followers: "Whoever eats My flesh and drinks My
blood has eternal life, and I will raise him up at the last day. For My flesh
is food indeed, and My blood is drink indeed. He who eats My flesh and
drinks My blood abides in Me, and I in him" (John 6:54–56). What does it
mean to be "in Christ"? He explains: "If you keep My commandments, you
will abide in My love, just as I have kept My Father's commandments and
abide in His love" (John 15:10).

To be in Christ means to abide in His love, which we do when we keep
His commandments. By the same token, "Christ in you" means love for
Christ dwells in you. "Eating His flesh and drinking His blood" is obviously
not to be taken literally. Christ pointed out that He meant we are to eat
His words, which are "spirit, and ... life" (John 6:63). Again, Christ really
means we are to accept those words of His by faith, which leads to our
salvation and results in our love for and obedience to Him (see Rom. 3:31).

Permit me to illustrate these concepts with an example. There is a sense
in which I am in my wife, and she is in me. One day, my wife decided some
bushes in our front yard were too large and we needed to remove them. She
requested that I do the removal. It turned out to be hard and sweaty work,
but I gladly did it because I love her. In a real sense, she was in me removing
those bushes. She was prompting my actions. For this to work, I had to be
humble enough to put her interests and opinion before my own. As Paul
said, "love does not parade itself, is not puffed up," and "does not seek its
own" (1 Cor. 13:4, 5).

It is important to understand the scope of Christ's words. He clearly
endorsed the words written by Moses: "Man shall not live by bread alone,
but by every word that proceeds from the mouth of God" (Matt. 4:4; see
Deut. 8:3). In the parable of the sower, the seed is the word of God (see Mark
4:14), which is pictured as growing and producing a harvest in those who
make room for it. Christ, in interceding with His Father for His followers,
prayed, "Sanctify them by Your truth. Your word is truth" (John 17:17).

Paul stated, "All Scripture *is* given by inspiration of God, and *is* profitable for doctrine, for reproof, for correction, for instruction in righteousness, that the man of God may be complete, thoroughly equipped for every good work" (2 Tim. 3:16, 17).

Christ offers us the privilege of walking with Him. "Come to Me, all you who labor and are heavy laden, and I will give you rest. Take My yoke upon you and learn from Me, for I am gentle and lowly in heart, and you will find rest for your souls. For My yoke is easy and My burden is light" (Matt. 11:28–30). If we accept Christ's yoke, we are then yoked with Him, and we must necessarily walk together. If we are in Christ and He is in us, this will happen naturally.

Paul expressed the result: "I have been crucified with Christ; it is no longer I who live, but Christ lives in me; and the *life* which I now live in the flesh I live by faith in the Son of God, who loved me and gave Himself for me" (Gal. 2:20). In working with Christ, Paul had learned humility and gave all the credit for his success to Christ: "But God forbid that I should boast except in the cross of our Lord Jesus Christ, by whom the world has been crucified to me, and I to the world" (6:14). If Christ lives in us, we, too, will live a life governed by His word and focused on spreading the gospel to the world. He promises, "I am with you always, even to the end of the age" (Matt. 28:20).

At the beginning of the conference, the organizers warned us that people were regularly being mugged in Prague, and the police were not doing much to stop the problem.

If you are in Christ and Christ is in you, you are yoked with Him. God makes many promises to you that do not apply to those who do not fear Him. One of His promises specifies that because you put His kingdom first, you have no need to worry and should not worry about the necessities of life, such as food and clothing (see Matt. 6:25–34). Additionally, God promises that events affecting you that may seem negative will be harnessed for your good: "And we know that all things work together for good to those who love God, to those who are the called according to His purpose" (Rom. 8:28).

I have experienced God's protecting care. In 2007, I attended the Association for Computational Linguistics Conference, held in Prague, Czech Republic. I attended as part of my professional duties since some of my work was presented in the associated BioNLP workshop. At the beginning of the conference, the organizers warned us that people were regularly being mugged in Prague, and the police were not doing much to stop the problem. We were urged to be careful, travel with a group, and avoid eye contact if in a threatening situation. The main conference ended on a Saturday, and the BioNLP workshop was on the following day.

Saturday morning, I got up at 5 a.m., as is my custom. I would keep the Sabbath holy and not attend the conference sessions that day. I spent some time reading my Bible and then thought it would be good to get out and walk in the early morning air. I wanted to go to the nearby metro station and see if I could figure out how to get to the Jan Hus Memorial. I knew the path that led to the metro. I headed off across a field, then along a road, and eventually down a street lined by houses, over a small footbridge, and arrived at the metro. No one was at the station, and nothing there was written in English, so I started on the path back to the hotel. When I had crossed the footbridge and arrived at the street lined with houses, everything was as quiet as when I had left it. No one was in sight.

Suddenly, all four doors of one of the cars along the street flew open, and out jumped four men. I did not stop walking, but this sent a chill up my spine. However, no sooner did these men jump out of the car then they proceeded to act as though no harm was intended. One stood by the car, three walked across the street, and one of those walked up to the entrance of one of the houses, which looked like it was also a business; he acted like he was seeking to enter. Of the other two, one stood near the road, and the biggest man proceeded to walk at a leisurely pace on the sidewalk in the direction I was heading. I continued to walk briskly, and when I caught up to the big man, I stepped into the street and walked past him. No one said a word. I don't know what they saw that changed their minds, but as far as I could see, I would have been an easy victim. I thanked God for His protection.

Ellen White pointed to a third benefit for those yoked with Christ:

> The love which Christ diffuses through the whole being is a vitalizing power. Every vital part—the brain, the heart, the nerves—it touches with healing. By it the highest energies of the being are aroused to activity. It frees the soul from the guilt and sorrow, the anxiety and care, that crush the life forces. With it come serenity and composure. It implants in the soul joy that nothing earthly can destroy,—joy in the Holy Spirit,—health-giving, life-giving joy. (*The Ministry of Healing*, p. 115)

With this, Paul agrees: "But if the Spirit of Him who raised Jesus from the dead dwells in you, He who raised Christ from the dead will also give life to your mortal bodies through His Spirit who dwells in you" (Rom. 8:11).

The Power

By His word, God created our world and all the life in it (see Gen. 1). Likewise, by His word, He created the heavens with their unnumbered stars and galaxies (see Ps. 33:6, 9). His word is powerful, even when spoken by His prophets. God demonstrated this to Ezekiel by instructing him to prophesy to a large collection of dry bones, that they should live, and they returned to life (see 37:1–14).

Notwithstanding, the power of God's word is mostly available through the prayer of faith. We are told that Joshua spoke to God (prayer) and then (inspired by God) commanded, "Sun, stand still over Gibeon; and Moon, in the Valley of Aijalon" (Josh. 10:12), and they obeyed! Likewise, Christ instructed, "For assuredly, I say to you, if you have faith as a mustard seed, you will say to this mountain, 'Move from here to there,' and it will move; and nothing will be impossible for you" (Matt. 17:20).

To experience the power of God, we must understand the prayer of faith. Ellen White emphasized the importance of this knowledge: "Prayer and faith are closely allied, and they need to be studied together. In the prayer of faith there is a divine science; it is a science that everyone who would make his lifework a success must understand" (1903, p. 257).

The first thing we need to understand is that God will not hear one who does not fear Him: "If I regard iniquity in my heart, the Lord will not hear" (Ps. 66:18); "The LORD is far from the wicked, but He hears the prayer of the righteous" (Prov. 15:29). "One who turns away his ear from hearing the law, even his prayer is an abomination" (28:9). God does not regard the prayers of those who seek to hide evil under a cloak of piety: "Indeed you fast for strife and debate, and to strike with the fist of wickedness. You will not fast as *you do* this day, to make your voice heard on high" (Isaiah 58:4); those "who devour widows' houses, and for a pretense make long prayers. These will receive greater condemnation" (Mark 12:40). In Christ's parable of the Pharisee and tax collector who went up to the temple to pray, it was not the proud Pharisee who benefited but the humble tax collector who went home justified (see Luke 18:10–14).

The key to answered prayer is to pray in harmony with God's will: "Now this is the confidence that we have in Him, that if we ask anything according to His will, He hears us. And if we know that He hears us, whatever we ask, we know that we have the petitions that we have asked of Him" (1 John 5:14, 15). Christ tied effective prayer to work for God: "Most assuredly, I say to you, he who believes in Me, the works that I do he will do also; and greater *works* than these he will do, because I go to My Father. And whatever you ask in My name, that I will do, that the Father may be glorified in the Son. If you ask anything in My name, I will do *it*" (John 14:12–14).

Praying in Christ's name cannot mean simply mouthing the phrase "in Jesus' name." It must mean we have evidence that Christ endorses what we request. This is supported by Christ's own statement: "If you abide in Me, and My words abide in you, you will ask what you desire, and it shall be done for you. By this My Father is glorified, that you bear much fruit; so you will be My disciples" (15:7, 8). Christ's words contain His promises, which we can present in our prayers.

When we have prayed in accordance with God's will, we must then exercise faith: "Now faith is the substance of things hoped for, the evidence of things not seen. For by it the elders obtained a *good* testimony. By faith we understand that the worlds were framed by the word of God, so that the things which are seen were not made of things which are visible" (Heb. 11:1–3). Faith is not guessing. It is fair treatment of the evidence (i.e., giving the evidence its proper weight). The evidence is the substance of our hopes (i.e., it is what we now have and can see).

God means we should have confidence in His promises, and He is displeased if we do not: "But without faith *it is* impossible to please *Him,* for he who comes to God must believe that He is, and *that* He is a rewarder of those who diligently seek Him" (verse 6). "If any of you lacks wisdom, let him ask of God, who gives to all liberally and without reproach, and it will be given to him. But let him ask in faith, with no doubting, for he who doubts is like a wave of the sea driven and tossed by the wind. For let not that man suppose that he will receive anything from the Lord" (James 1:5–7).

As Ellen White stated, "Christ says, 'What things soever ye desire, when ye pray, believe that ye receive them, and ye shall have them.' Mark 11:24. He makes it plain that our asking must be according to God's will; we must ask for the things that He has promised, and whatever we receive must be used in doing His will. The conditions met, the promise is unequivocal" (1903, p. 257).

God's purpose in this world is salvation for all who are willing to be saved. God's power for this purpose is in His word. Christ said, "Sanctify them by Your truth. Your word is truth" (John 17:17). Paul saw God's power as concentrated in the gospel: "For I am not ashamed of the gospel of Christ, for it is the power of God to salvation for everyone who believes, for the Jew first and also for the Greek" (Rom. 1:16).

For Peter, the power is found in the knowledge of God:

> Grace and peace be multiplied to you in the knowledge of God and of Jesus our Lord, as His divine power has given to us all things that *pertain* to life and godliness, through the knowledge of Him who called us by glory and virtue, by which have been given to us exceedingly great and precious promises, that through these you may be partakers of the divine nature, having escaped the corruption *that is* in the world through lust. (2 Peter 1:2–4)

Salvation from sin is ours to accept by faith, but we must trust God's promises. One great promise is "If we confess our sins, He is faithful and just to forgive us *our* sins and to cleanse us from all unrighteousness" (1 John 1:9). Another is the promise of the Holy Spirit: "If you then, being evil, know how to give good gifts to your children, how much more will *your* heavenly Father give the Holy Spirit to those who ask Him!" (Luke 11:13). In these two promises, the benefits of the new covenant are made available to us and all who are willing to claim them by faith.

Ellen White provided insights regarding the power of God as it pertains to us:

> The whole Bible is a manifestation of Christ. It is our only source of power. (*Gospel Workers*, p. 250)

> So with all the promises of God's word. In them He is speaking to us individually, speaking as directly as if we could listen to His voice. It is in these promises that Christ communicates to us His grace and power. They are leaves from that tree which is "for the healing of the nations." Revelation 22:2. Received, assimilated, they are to be the strength of the character, the inspiration and sustenance of the life. Nothing else can have such healing power. Nothing besides can impart the courage and faith which give vital energy to the whole being. (*The Ministry of Healing*, p. 122)

If Christ has promised, and we know God's will is for us to fulfill the conditions of the promise and claim its benefits by faith yet do not do this, that is a sinful lack of faith. "But the cowardly, unbelieving, abominable … and all liars shall have their part in the lake which burns with fire and brimstone, which is the second death" (Rev. 21:8). However, we do not always know what the will of God is. How shall we pray in that situation? Christ's model prayer begins with the words, "Our Father in heaven, hallowed be Your name. Your kingdom come. Your will be done on earth as *it is* in heaven" (Luke 11:2). Sometimes, we must simply pray that God's will be done. Before the cross, Christ prayed for some other path if possible: "O My Father, if it is possible, let this cup pass from Me; nevertheless, not as I will, but as You *will*" (Matt. 26:39).

For those inclined to boast about what they planned to do in the future, James counseled, "Instead you *ought* to say, 'If the Lord wills, we shall live and do this or that'" (4:15). In many things, including prayers for the sick, it is appropriate to pray for what we hope but leave the outcome to God's will: "Be anxious for nothing, but in everything by prayer and supplication, with thanksgiving, let your requests be made known to God; and the peace of God, which surpasses all understanding, will guard your hearts and minds through Christ Jesus" (Phil. 4:6, 7).

I have seen my prayers answered many times. The most dramatic instance occurred in 1961, while I was a freshman at Pacific Union College. My eldest brother Dave had gotten married and gone on to graduate school at UC Berkeley. Dave had just acquired a Chevy Corvair and loaned it to my other brother Irv. Irv, then a senior at PUC, was to drive his girlfriend and a friend of hers along with me home from college for the Thanksgiving holiday. Irv was a good driver but had no experience driving a Corvair. The engine was in the rear of the car, so we loaded our bags under the front hood. As we stopped before turning onto the main highway that led down into the Napa Valley, I felt strongly impressed that I needed to pray.

When traveling with my parents, we always prayed before major travel. I asked my brother to pause while I prayed a short prayer for protection on our trip. We started on our trip and, within less than a mile, reached a long, curvy stretch of the two-lane highway. We were on the inside of the curve, and the back of the car began to slide out into the opposite lane. That would not have been so serious, but a car was traveling in the opposite direction and getting closer to us. Irv had no choice but to steer hard to the right.

When he did this, the right front tire caught a tar ridge at the edge of the road. The car immediately flipped. What motion the car took, I do not know. I felt a spinning sensation, and then we were all sitting in our places in the car, which was now down off the road and sitting between two small trees. (This was before the days of seat belts.) The windshield was missing, but there was no other obvious damage. The friend complained of some neck pain, which I don't believe proved serious. No one else complained of any injury. The trip was cancelled, but we had much for which to be thankful. I was strongly convinced that God had impressed me to pray and had answered my prayer. The Corvair eventually gained a reputation as very unsafe, initiated by activist and author Ralph Nader, but the maker, Edward N. Cole, strongly contested the claim.

The Apocalypse

God has a plan to end the world at Christ's second coming. Christ illustrated events we are to expect at that time with the parable of the wheat and tares (see Matt. 13:36–43). The tares represent the wicked who will be destroyed; the wheat, the righteous who will be taken to heaven. Before the end, an urgent warning will be given to the earth's inhabitants: "Behold, I will send you Elijah the prophet before the coming of the great and dreadful day of the LORD. And he will turn the hearts of the fathers to the children, and the hearts of the children to their fathers, lest I come and strike the earth with a curse" (Mal. 4:5, 6).

God's power will attend the warning. He will pour out the Holy Spirit on His people. There will also be warning signs on earth and in the heavens, and salvation will be available to those who repent (see Joel 2:28–32). While this prophecy was invoked to explain the day of Pentecost (Acts 2:16–21), the signs spoken of were still future at that time. We look for another fulfillment near the end. This fulfillment is described in Revelation 18:1–8, where Babylon's fall is proclaimed and those desiring salvation are urged to come out of her to escape her impending destruction.

Christ commanded His followers to "love one another as I have loved you" (John 15:12). He further pointed out that their witness would be effective if they loved one another:

> That they all may be one, as You, Father, *are* in Me, and I in You; that they also may be one in Us, that the world may believe that You sent Me. And the glory which You gave Me I have given them, that they may be one just as We are one: I in them, and You in Me; that they may be made perfect in one, and that the world may know that You have sent Me, and have loved them as You have loved Me. (John 17:21–23)

The love the members of God's church have for each other is to be the proof to the world that we have a message that is true and crucial to their salvation. Thus, Paul can write to Timothy, "*I write* so that you may know how you ought to conduct yourself in the house of God, which is the church of the living God, the pillar and ground of the truth" (1 Tim. 3:15).

To love others as Christ has loved us is a high standard. Unselfish love was clearly demonstrated in Moses, Jonathan, and John the Baptist and must have been present in all who truly served God. After Christ's death, His followers were influenced by an unselfish spirit. On the day of Pentecost, they were all in one accord (see Acts 2:1). As many joined the church, this selfless behavior continued: "Now all who believed were together, and had all things in common, and sold their possessions and goods, and divided them among all, as anyone had need. So continuing daily with one accord in the temple, and breaking bread from house to house, they ate their food with gladness and simplicity of heart" (Acts 2:44–46—Unfortunately, near the end of the first century, when John was writing Revelation, this love was no longer a driving force in the Ephesian church. They had ceased to be a light to their community [see Revelation 2:5]. Unloving behavior is sin, and repentance was needed).

In what practical way can we come to have unselfish love for each other in our day? Ellen White laid out in clear lines what we need: "We need not begin by *trying* to love one another. The love of Christ in the heart is what is needed. When self is submerged in Christ, true love springs forth spontaneously" (1915, p. 497). What does it mean that "self is submerged in Christ?" Again, she provided an answer:

> When self is submerged in Christ, true love springs forth spontaneously. It is not an emotion or an impulse but a decision of a sanctified will. It consists not in feeling, but in the transformation of the whole heart, soul, and character, which is dead to self and alive unto God. Our Lord and Saviour asks us to give ourselves to Him. Surrendering self to God is all He requires, giving ourselves to Him to be employed as He sees fit. Until we come to this point of surrender, we shall not work happily, usefully, or successfully anywhere. (*Mind, Character, and Personality*, vol. 1, p. 206)

Here, we see the objective, but not how to get there. Some things, we cannot do for ourselves:

None but God can subdue the pride of man's heart. We cannot save ourselves. We cannot regenerate ourselves. In the heavenly courts there will be no song sung, To me that loved myself, and washed myself, redeemed myself, unto me be glory and honor, blessing and praise. But this is the keynote of the song that is sung by many here in this world. They do not know what it means to be meek and lowly in heart; and they do not mean to know this, if they can avoid it. The whole gospel is comprised in learning of Christ, His meekness and lowliness. (*Testimonies to Ministers and Gospel Workers*, p. 456)

The power to transform us is in God's Word, which we must study, and in its promises, which we are to claim by faith. Then by faith, we can rest in the assurance that God's purposes will be carried out in our lives. "Beloved, I beg *you* as sojourners and pilgrims, abstain from fleshly lusts which war against the soul" (1 Peter 2:11). "*Be* kindly affectionate to one another with brotherly love, in honor giving preference to one another; not lagging in diligence, fervent in spirit, serving the Lord" (Rom. 12:10, 11). "*Let* nothing *be done* through selfish ambition or conceit, but in lowliness of mind let each esteem others better than himself. Let each of you look out not only for his own interests, but also for the interests of others" (Phil. 2:3, 4).

Since these verses express God's will for us, we can treat them as promises and ask God to make them effective in our lives (see 1 John 5:14, 15). By faith, we will be able to carry them out in practice. "The creative energy that called the worlds into existence is in the word of God. This word imparts power; it begets life. Every command is a promise; accepted by the will, received into the soul, it brings with it the life of the Infinite One. It transforms the nature and re-creates the soul in the image of God" (White 1903, p. 126). Through God's power, by faith, a loving heart is within the reach of His people.

In the days of Christ's apostles, signs and wonders gave impetus to the gospel message:

And through the hands of the apostles many signs and wonders were done among the people. And they were all with one accord in Solomon's Porch. Yet none of the rest dared join them, but the people esteemed them highly. And believers were increasingly added to the Lord, multitudes of both men and women, so that they brought the sick out into the streets and laid *them* on beds and couches, that at least the shadow of Peter passing by might fall on some of them. Also a multitude gathered from the surrounding cities to Jerusalem, bringing sick people and those who were tormented by unclean spirits, and they were all healed. (Acts 5:12–16)

Now God worked unusual miracles by the hands of Paul, so that even handkerchiefs or aprons were brought from his body to the sick, and the diseases left them and the evil spirits went out of them. (Acts 19:11, 12)

Had not God's people loved each other, there would have been no power in their witness and no value in signs and wonders to attract people to the message. When God's people again demonstrate love for each other, this will be the time when His power will be displayed to attract others to His message and hasten the message to all the world.

> *When God's people again demonstrate love for each other, this will be the time when His power will be displayed to hasten the message to all the world.*

God has a work for His people to do for the world, and if they will work in harmony with one another and with heaven, He will demonstrate His power in their behalf as He did for His first disciples on the day of Pentecost. (White, *The Faith I Live By*, p. 332)

Search heaven and earth, and there is no truth revealed more powerful than that which is made manifest in works of mercy to those who need our sympathy and aid. This is the truth as it is in Jesus. When those who profess the name of Christ shall practice the principles of the golden rule, the same power will attend the gospel as in apostolic times. (White, *Thoughts from the Mount of Blessing*, p. 137)

What has looked like an impossible task from a human perspective will happen quickly. "And this gospel of the kingdom will be preached in all the world as a witness to all the nations, and then the end will come" (Matt. 24:14).

Bibliography

Aagaard, P., C. Suetta, P. Caserotti, S.P. Magnusson, and M. Kjaer. "Role of the nervous system in sarcopenia and muscle atrophy with aging: strength training as a countermeasure." *Scandinavian Journal of Medicine & Science in Sports* 20, no. 1 (2010): pp. 49–64.

Abbasi, J. "Coconut Oil's Health Halo a Mirage, Clinical Trials Suggest." *JAMA* 323, no. 16 (2020): pp. 1540–1541.

Abbasi, J. "TMAO and Heart Disease: The New Red Meat Risk?" *JAMA* 321, no. 22, (2019): pp. 2149–2151.

Abdelhamid AS, Brown TJ, Brainard JS, Biswas P, Thorpe GC, Moore HJ, et al. "Omega-3 fatty acids for the primary and secondary prevention of cardiovascular disease." *Cochrane Database of System Reviews* 3, no. 3 (2020): CD003177.

Adafer, R., W. Messaadi, M. Meddahi, A. Patey, A. Haderbache, S. Bayen, et al. "Food Timing, Circadian Rhythm and Chrononutrition: A Systematic Review of Time-Restricted Eating's Effects on Human Health." *Nutrients* 12, no. 12 (2020): p. 3770.

"Adult Obesity Facts." Centers for Disease Control and Prevention. https://www.cdc.gov/obesity/data/adult.html (last reviewed May 17, 2022).

Aebersold, R., J.N. Agar, I.J. Amster, M.S. Baker, C.R. Bertozzi, E.S. Boja, et al. "How many human proteoforms are there?" *Nature Chemical Biology* 14, n. 3 (2018): pp. 206–214.

Ahima, R.S., and D.A. Antwi. "Brain regulation of appetite and satiety." *Endocrinology and Metabolism Clinics of North America* 37, no. 4 (2008): pp. 811–823.

Ainsworth, B.E., W.L. Haskell, A.S. Leon, D.R. Jacobs Jr., H.J. Montoye, J.F. Sallis, et al. "Compendium of physical activities: classification of energy costs of human physical activities." *Medicine & Science in Sports & Exercise* 25, no. 1 (1993): pp. 71–80.

Almohammed, O.A., A.A. Alsalem, A.A. Almangour, L.H. Alotaibi, M.S. Al Yami, and L. Lai. "Antidepressants and health-related quality of life (HRQoL) for patients with depression: Analysis of the medical expenditure panel survey from the United States." *PLOS One* 17, no. 4 (2022): e0265928.

Arem, H., S.C. Moore, A. Patel, P. Hartge, A. Berrington de Gonzalez, K. Visvanathan, et al. "Leisure time physical activity and mortality: a detailed pooled analysis of the dose-response relationship." *JAMA Internal Medicine* 175, no. 6 (2015): pp. 959–967.

Atroszko, P.A., Z. Demetrovics, and M.D. Griffiths. "Work Addiction, Obsessive-Compulsive Personality Disorder, Burn-Out, and Global Burden of Disease: Implications from the ICD-11." *International Journal of Environmental Research and Public Health* 17, no. 2 (2020): p. 660.

Bacchetti, T., I. Turco, A. Urbano, C. Morresi, and G. Ferretti. "Relationship of fruit and vegetable intake to dietary antioxidant capacity and markers of oxidative stress: A sex-related study." *Nutrition* 61 (2019): pp. 164–172.

Baer, D.J., W.V. Rumpler, C.W. Miles, and G.C. Fahey Jr. "Dietary fiber decreases the metabolizable energy content and nutrient digestibility of mixed diets fed to humans." *Journal of Nutrition* 127, no. 4 (1997): pp. 579–586.

Baker, V.R. "Catastrophism and uniformitarianism: logical roots and current relevance in geology." *Geological Society, London, Special Publications* 143 (1998): pp. 171–182.

Baker, V.R. "The Channeled Scabland: A Retrospective." *Annual Review of Earth and Planetary Sciences* 37 (2009): pp. 393–411.

Bannai, A., and A. Tamakoshi. "The association between long working hours and health: a systematic review of epidemiological evidence." *Scandinavian Journal of Work, Environment & Health* 40, no. 1 (2014): pp. 5–18.

Bansal, N., M. Hudda, R.A. Payne, D.J. Smith, D. Kessler, and N. Wiles. "Antidepressant use and risk of adverse outcomes: population-based cohort study." *BJPsych Open* 8, no. 5 (2022): e164.

Barnard, Neal. *Dr. Neal Barnard's Program for Reversing Diabetes: The Scientifically Proven System for Reversing Diabetes Without Drugs.* Emmaus, PA: Rodale, Inc., 2018.

Beare, J.L. "Fatty Acid Composition of Food Fats." *The Journal of Agricultural and Food Chemistry* 10, no. 2 (1962): pp. 120–123.

Beaulieu, K., P. Oustric, S. Alkahtani, M. Alhussain, H. Pedersen, J.S. Quist, et al. "Impact of Meal Timing and Chronotype on Food Reward and Appetite Control in Young Adults." *Nutrients* 12, no. 5 (2020): p. 1506.

Beecher, H.K. "Surgery as placebo. A quantitative study of bias." *JAMA* 176, no. 13 (1961): pp. 1102–1107.

Behe, Michael. *Darwin devolves: the new science about DNA that challenges evolution.* New York: HarperOne, 2019.

Bellesi, M., D. Bushey, M. Chini, G. Tononi, and C. Cirelli. "Contribution of sleep to the repair of neuronal DNA double-strand breaks: evidence from flies and mice." *Scientific Reports* 6, no. 36804 (2016).

Bentley, Jeanine. *U.S. Trends in Food Availability and a Dietary Assessment of Loss-Adjusted Food Availability, 1970–2014.* United States Department of Agriculture, 2017.

Benzell, S.G., and K. Cooke. "A Network of Thrones: Kinship and Conflict in Europe, 1495–1918." *American Economic Journal: Applied Economics* 13, no. 3 (2021): pp. 102–133.

Berkel, J., and F. de Waard. "Mortality pattern and life expectancy of Seventh-Day Adventists in the Netherlands." *International Journal of Epidemiology* 12, n. 4 (1983): pp. 455–459.

Berlinski, David. *The Devil's Delusion: Atheism and Its Scientific Pretensions.* New York: Basic Books, 2009.

Bianconi, E., A. Piovesan, F. Facchin, A. Beraudi, R. Casadei, F. Frabetti, et al. "An estimation of the number of cells in the human body." Annals Human Biology 40, no. 6 (2013): pp. 463–471.

Bielefeldt, A.O., P.B. Danborg, and P.C. Gotzsche. "Precursors to suicidality and violence on antidepressants: systematic review of trials in adult healthy volunteers." *Journal of the Royal Society of Medicine* 109, no. 10 (2016): pp. 381–392.

Bishop, S.R., M. Lau, S. Shapiro, L. Carlson, N.D. Anderson, J. Carmody, Z.V. Segal, S. Abbey, M. Speca, D. Velting, and G. Devins. "Mindfulness:

A proposed operational definition." Clinical Psychology: Science and Practice 11, no. 3 (2004): pp. 230–241.

Blais, C.A., R.M. Pangborn, N.O. Borhani, M.F. Ferrell, R.J. Prineas, and B. Laing. "Effect of dietary sodium restriction on taste responses to sodium chloride: a longitudinal study." *American Journal of Clinical Nutrition* 44, no. 2 (1986): pp. 232–243.

Bluher, M. "Obesity: global epidemiology and pathogenesis." *Nature Reviews Endocrinology* 15, no. 5 (2019): pp. 288–298.

Boivin, D.B., P. Boudreau, and A. Kosmadopoulos. "Disturbance of the Circadian System in Shift Work and Its Health Impact." *Journal of Biological Rhythms* 37, no. 1 (2022): pp. 3–28.

Borbely, A.A., S. Daan, A. Wirz-Justice, and T. Deboer. "The two-process model of sleep regulation: a reappraisal." *Journal of Sleep Research* 25, no. 2 (2016): pp. 131–143.

Bray, G.A., J.C. Lovejoy, M. Most-Windhauser, S.R. Smith, J. Volaufova, Y. Denkins, et al. "A 9-mo randomized clinical trial comparing fat-substituted and fat-reduced diets in healthy obese men: the Ole Study." *American Journal of Clinical Nutrition* 76, no. 5 (2002): pp. 928–934.

Brondel, L., M. Romer, V. Van Wymelbeke, P. Walla, T. Jiang, L. Deecke, et al. "Sensory-specific satiety with simple foods in humans: no influence of BMI?" *International Journal of Obesity* 31, no. 6 (2007): pp. 987–995.

Brown, T.J., J. Brainard, F. Song, X. Wang, A. Abdelhamid, L. Hooper, et al. "Omega-3, omega-6, and total dietary polyunsaturated fat for prevention and treatment of type 2 diabetes mellitus: systematic review and meta-analysis of randomised controlled trials." *BMJ* 366 (2019): l4697.

Buckalew, L.W., and K.E. Coffield. "An investigation of drug expectancy as a function of capsule color and size and preparation form." *Journal of Clinical Psychopharmacology* 2, no. 4 (1982): pp. 245–248.

Burckhardt, M., M. Herke, T. Wustmann, S. Watzke, G. Langer, and A. Fink. "Omega-3 fatty acids for the treatment of dementia." *Cochrane Database of System Reviews* 4 (2016): CD009002.

Burns, David. *Feeling Good: The New Mood Therapy*. New York: HarperCollins, 1980.

Cappuccio, F.P., L. D'Elia, P. Strazzullo, and M.A. Miller. "Quantity and quality of sleep and incidence of type 2 diabetes: a systematic review and meta-analysis." *Diabetes Care* 33, no. 2 (2010): pp. 414–420.

Capuano, E., T. Oliviero, V. Fogliano, and N. Pellegrini. "Role of the food matrix and digestion on calculation of the actual energy content of food." *Nutrition Reviews* 76, no. 4 (2018): pp. 274–289.

Carter, J.P., and J. Brown. "Dr. Cupp's simple approach to weight loss." *Journal of the Louisiana State Medical Society* 137, no. 6 (1985): pp. 35–38.

Caspi, A., R.M. Houts, A. Ambler, A. Danese, M.L. Elliott, A. Hariri, et al. "Longitudinal Assessment of Mental Health Disorders and Comorbidities Across 4 Decades Among Participants in the Dunedin Birth Cohort Study." *JAMA Network Open* 3, no. 4 (2020): e203221.

Caspi, A., and T.E. Moffitt. "All for One and One for All: Mental Disorders in One Dimension." *American Journal of Psychiatry* 175, no. 9 (2018): pp. 831–844.

Catenacci, V.A., L. Odgen, S. Phelan, J.G. Thomas, J. Hill, R.R. Wing, et al. "Dietary habits and weight maintenance success in high versus low exercisers in the National Weight Control Registry." *Journal of Physical Activity and Health* 11, no. 8 (2014): pp. 1540–1548.

Celis-Morales, C.A., P. Welsh, D.M. Lyall, L. Steell, F. Petermann, J. Anderson, et al. "Associations of grip strength with cardiovascular, respiratory, and cancer outcomes and all cause mortality: prospective cohort study of half a million UK Biobank participants." *BMJ* 361 (2018): k1651.

Chalder, T., K.A. Goldsmith, P.D. White, M. Sharpe, and A.R. Pickles. "Rehabilitative therapies for chronic fatigue syndrome: a secondary mediation analysis of the PACE trial." *The Lancet Psychiatry* 2, no. 2 (2015): pp. 141–152.

Chan, J., S.F. Knutsen, G.G. Blix, J.W. Lee, and G.E. Fraser. "Water, other fluids, and fatal coronary heart disease: the Adventist Health Study." *American Journal of Epidemiology* 155, no. 9 (2002): pp. 827–833.

Chavez, M.N., and K.K. Rigg. "Nutritional implications of opioid use disorder: A guide for drug treatment providers." *Psychology of Addictive Behaviors* 34, no. 6 (2020): pp. 699–707.

Chen, C., X. Li, Y. Su, Z. You, R. Wan, and K. Hong. "Adherence with cardiovascular medications and the outcomes in patients with coronary arterial disease: 'Real-world' evidence." *Clinical Cardiology* 45, no. 12 (2022): pp. 1220–1228.

Chen, F., M. Du, J.B. Blumberg, K.K. Ho Chui, M. Ruan, G. Rogers, et al. "Association Among Dietary Supplement Use, Nutrient Intake, and Mortality Among U.S. Adults: A Cohort Study." *Annals of Internal Medicine* 170, no. 9 (2019): pp. 604–613.

Chen, X., Z. Zhang, H. Yang, P. Qiu, H. Wang, F. Wang, et al. "Consumption of ultra-processed foods and health outcomes: a systematic review of epidemiological studies." *Nutrition Journal* 19, no. 1 (2020): p. 86.

Chowdhury, R., H. Khan, E. Heydon, A. Shroufi, S. Fahimi, C. Moore, et al. "Adherence to cardiovascular therapy: a meta-analysis of prevalence and clinical consequences." *European Heart Journal* 34, no. 38 (2013): pp. 2940–2948.

Chung, H.K., J.H. Kim, A. Choi, C.W. Ahn, Y.S. Kim, and J.S. Nam. "Antioxidant-Rich Dietary Intervention Improves Cardiometabolic Profiles and Arterial Stiffness in Elderly Koreans with Metabolic Syndrome." *Yonsei Medical Journal* 63, no. 1 (2022): pp. 26–33.

Churchill, Winston "Hansard Committee Debate." July 29, 1941, pp. cc1273–1330.

Cifuentes, L., and A. Acosta. "Homeostatic regulation of food intake." *Clinics and Research in Hepatology and Gastroenterology* 46, no. 2 (2022): p. 101794.

Cipriani A, Furukawa TA, Salanti G, Chaimani A, Atkinson LZ, Ogawa Y, et al. "Comparative efficacy and acceptability of 21 antidepressant drugs for the acute treatment of adults with major depressive disorder: a systematic review and network meta-analysis." *The Lancet* 391, no. 10128 (2018): pp. 1357–1366.

Clayton, D.J., and L.J. James. "The effect of breakfast on appetite regulation, energy balance and exercise performance." *Proceedings of the Nutrition Society* 75, no. 3 (2016): pp. 319–327.

Cocate, P.G., A.J. Natali, A. Oliveira, G.Z. Longo, R.C.G. Alfenas, M.C.G. Peluzio, et al. "Fruit and vegetable intake and related nutrients are associated with oxidative stress markers in middle-aged men." *Nutrition* 30, no. 6 (2014): pp. 660–665.

Cohen, S., D. Janicki-Deverts, W.J. Doyle, G.E. Miller, E. Frank, B.S. Rabin, et al. "Chronic stress, glucocorticoid receptor resistance, inflammation, and disease risk." *Proceedings of the National Academy of Sciences of the United States of America* 109, no. 16 (2012): pp. 5995–5999.

Colak A, Akinci B, Diniz G, Turkon H, Ergonen F, Yalcin H, et al. "Postload hyperglycemia is associated with increased subclinical inflammation in patients with prediabetes." *Scandinavian Journal of Clinical & Laboratory Investigation* 73, no. 5 (2013): pp. 422–427.

Cook, D.B., S. VanRiper, R.J. Dougherty, J.B. Lindheimer, M.J. Falvo, Y. Chen, et al. "Cardiopulmonary, metabolic, and perceptual responses during exercise in Myalgic Encephalomyelitis/Chronic Fatigue Syndrome (ME/CFS): A Multi-site Clinical Assessment of ME/CFS (MCAM) sub-study." *PLOS One* 17, no. 3 (2022): e0265315.

Coon, Roger. *A Gift of Light.* 2nd ed. Hagerstown, MD: Review and Hearld Publishing Association, 1998.

Cowan, J., and C. Devine. "Food, eating, and weight concerns of men in recovery from substance addiction." *Appetite* 50, no. 1 (2008): pp. 33–42.

Cowan, R.L., I.K. Lyoo, S.M. Sung, K.H. Ahn, M.J. Kim, J. Hwang, et al. "Reduced cortical gray matter density in human MDMA (Ecstasy) users: a voxel-based morphometry study." *Drug and Alcohol Dependence* 72, no. 3 (2003): pp. 225–235.

Crippa, A., A. Discacciati, S.C. Larsson, A. Wolk, and N. Orsini. "Coffee consumption and mortality from all causes, cardiovascular disease, and cancer: a dose-response meta-analysis." *American Journal of Epidemiology* 180, no. 8 (2014): pp. 763–775.

Cuddy, T.F., J.S. Ramos, and L.C. Dalleck. "Reduced Exertion High-Intensity Interval Training is More Effective at Improving Cardiorespiratory Fitness and Cardiometabolic Health than Traditional Moderate-Intensity Continuous Training." *International Journal of Environmental Research and Public Health* 16, no. 3 (2019): p. 483.

D'Arcy, M.S. "Cell death: a review of the major forms of apoptosis, necrosis and autophagy." *Cell Biology International* 43, no. 6 (2019): pp. 582–592.

Daumann J, Koester P, Becker B, Wagner D, Imperati D, Gouzoulis-Mayfrank E, et al. "Medial prefrontal gray matter volume reductions in users of amphetamine-type stimulants revealed by combined tract-based spatial statistics and voxel-based morphometry." *NeuroImage* 54, no. 2 (2011): pp. 794–801.

David, A.R., A. Kershaw, and A. Heagerty. "Atherosclerosis and diet in ancient Egypt." *The Lancet* 375, no. 9716 (2010): pp. 718–719.

de Oliveira Otto, M.C., A. Alonso, D.H. Lee, G.L. Delclos, A.G. Bertoni, R. Jiang, et al. "Dietary intakes of zinc and heme iron from red meat, but not from other sources, are associated with greater risk of metabolic syndrome and cardiovascular disease." *Journal of Nutrition* 142, no. 3 (2012): pp. 526–533.

de Oliveira Otto, M.C., D. Mozaffarian, D. Kromhout, A.G. Bertoni, C.T. Sibley, D.R. Jacobs Jr., et al. "Dietary intake of saturated fat by food source and incident cardiovascular disease: the Multi-Ethnic Study of Atherosclerosis." *American Journal of Clinical Nutrition* 96, no. 2 (2012): pp. 397–404.

de Witte, M., A.D.S. Pinho, G.J. Stams, X. Moonen, A.E.R. Bos, and S. van Hooren. "Music therapy for stress reduction: a systematic review and meta-analysis." *Health Psychology Review* 16, no. 1 (2022): pp. 134–159.

Degens, Hans. "Human Ageing: Impact on Muscle Force and Power." Chap. 19 in *Muscle and Exercise Physiology*. Amsterdam: Elsevier Publishing, 2019.

Deguil, J., L. Pineau, E.C. Rowland Snyder, S. Dupont, L. Beney, A. Gil, et al. "Modulation of lipid-induced ER stress by fatty acid shape." *Traffic* 12, no. 3 (2011): pp. 349–362.

del Pozo, C.B., M. Ahmadi, I. Lee, and E. Stamatakis. "Prospective Associations of Daily Step Counts and Intensity With Cancer and Cardiovascular Disease Incidence and Mortality and All-Cause Mortality." *JAMA Internal Medicine* 182, no. 11 (2022): pp. 1139–1148.

Dement, William, and Christopher Vaughan. *The Promise of Sleep*. New York: Dell Publishing, 1999.

DeSilver, Drew. "What's on your table? How America's diet has changed over the decades." Pew Research Center. https://www.pewresearch.org/fact-tank/2016/12/13/whats-on-your-table-how-americas-diet-has-changed-over-the-decades, December 13, 2016.

Deumer, U.S., A. Varesi, V. Floris, G. Savioli, E. Mantovani, P. Lopez-Carrasco, et al. "Myalgic Encephalomyelitis/Chronic Fatigue Syndrome (ME/CFS): An Overview." *Journal of Clinical Medicine* 10, no. 20 (2021): p. 4786.

DiNicolantonio, J.J., S.C. Lucan, and J.H. O'Keefe. "The Evidence for Saturated Fat and for Sugar Related to Coronary Heart Disease." *Progress in Cardiovascular Diseases* 58, no. 5 (2016): pp. 464–472.

DiNicolantonio, J.J., and J.H. O'Keefe. "Good Fats versus Bad Fats: A Comparison of Fatty Acids in the Promotion of Insulin Resistance, Inflammation, and Obesity." *Missouri Medicine* 114, no. 4 (2017): pp. 303–307.

Doepker, C., N. Movva, S.S. Cohen, and D.S. Wikoff. "Benefit-risk of coffee consumption and all-cause mortality: A systematic review and disability adjusted life year analysis." *Food and Chemical Toxicology* 170 (2022): p. 113472.

Drouin-Chartier, J.P., A.J. Tremblay, J. Maltais-Giguere, A. Charest, L. Guinot, L.E. Rioux, et al. "Differential impact of the cheese matrix on the postprandial lipid response: a randomized, crossover, controlled trial." *American Journal of Clinical Nutrition* 106, no. 6 (2017): pp. 1358–1365.

DuBroff, R. "Cholesterol paradox: a correlate does not a surrogate make." *Journal of Evidence-Based Medicine* 22, no. 1 (2017): pp. 15–19.

DuBroff, R., and M. de Lorgeril. "Cholesterol confusion and statin controversy." *World Journal of Cardiology* 7, no. 7 (2015): pp. 404–409.

Duckert, L.G., and T.S. Rees. "Placebo effect in tinnitus management." *Otolaryngology—Head and Neck Surgery* 92, no. 6 (1984): pp. 697–699.

Duncan, K.H., J.A. Bacon, and R.L. Weinsier. "The effects of high and low energy density diets on satiety, energy intake, and eating time of obese and nonobese subjects." *American Journal of Clinical Nutrition* 37, no. 5 (1983): pp. 763–767.

"Eating, Diet, & Nutrition for Dumping Syndrome." National Institute of Diabetes and Digestive and Kidney Diseases. https://www.niddk.nih.gov/health-information/digestive-diseases/dumping-syndrome/eating-diet-nutrition (last reviewed January 2019).

Eguchi, K., I. Manabe, Y. Oishi-Tanaka, M. Ohsugi, N. Kono, F. Ogata, et al. "Saturated fatty acid and TLR signaling link beta cell dysfunction and islet inflammation." *Cell Metabolism* 15, no. 4 (2012): pp. 518–533.

Elgaddal, N., E.A. Kramarow, and C. Reuben. "Physical Activity Among Adults Aged 18 and Over: United States, 2020." Centers for Disease Control and Prevention. https://www.cdc.gov/nchs/products/databriefs/db443.htm, August 2022.

Elizabeth, L., P. Machado, M. Zinocker, P. Baker, and M. Lawrence. "Ultra-Processed Foods and Health Outcomes: A Narrative Review." *Nutrients* 12, no. 7 (2020): p. 1955.

Ellis, P.R., C.W. Kendall, Y. Ren, C. Parker, J.F. Pacy, K.W. Waldron, et al. "Role of cell walls in the bioaccessibility of lipids in almond seeds." *American Journal of Clinical Nutrition* 80, no. 3 (2004): pp. 604–613.

Ely, A.V., and R.R. Wetherill. "Reward and inhibition in obesity and cigarette smoking: Neurobiological overlaps and clinical implications." *Physiology & Behavior* 260 (2022): p. 114049.

Embling, R., A.E. Pink, J. Gatzemeier, M. Price M, M.D. Lee, and L.L. Wilkinson. "Effect of food variety on intake of a meal: a systematic review and meta-analysis." *American Journal of Clinical Nutrition* 113, no. 3 (2021): pp. 716–741.

Erbay Dalli, O., C. Bozkurt, and Y. Yildirim. "The effectiveness of music interventions on stress response in intensive care patients: A systematic review and meta-analysis." *Journal of Clinical Nursing* 32, nos. 11, 12 (2022): pp. 2827–2845.

Ersche, K.D., A. Barnes, P.S. Jones, S. Morein-Zamir, T.W. Robbins, and E.T. Bullmore. "Abnormal structure of frontostriatal brain systems is associated with aspects of impulsivity and compulsivity in cocaine dependence." *Brain* 134, pt. 7 (2011): pp. 2013–2024.

Esposito, K., F. Nappo, R. Marfella, G. Giugliano, F. Giugliano, M. Ciotola, et al. "Inflammatory cytokine concentrations are acutely increased by hyperglycemia in humans: role of oxidative stress." *Circulation* 106, no. 16 (2002): pp. 2067–2072.

Esselstyn Jr., C.B, G. Gendy, J. Doyle, M. Golubic, and M.F. Roizen. "A way to reverse CAD?" *The Journal of Family Practice* 63, no. 7 (2014): pp. 356–364b.

Feltenstein, M.W., R.E. See, and R.A. Fuchs. "Neural Substrates and Circuits of Drug Addiction." *Cold Spring Harbor Perspectives in Medicine* 11, no. 4, (2021): a039628.

Ference, B.A., J.J.P. Kastelein, H.N. Ginsberg, M.J. Chapman, S.J. Nicholls, K.K. Ray, et al. "Association of Genetic Variants Related to CETP Inhibitors and Statins With Lipoprotein Levels and Cardiovascular Risk." *JAMA* 318, no. 10 (2017): pp. 947–956.

Fernandez-Mendoza, J., F. He, A.N. Vgontzas, D. Liao, and E.O. Bixler. "Interplay of Objective Sleep Duration and Cardiovascular and Cerebrovascular Diseases on Cause-Specific Mortality." *Journal of the American Heart Association* 8, no. 20 (2019): p. e013043.

Ferreira, A., J.P. Castro, J.P. Andrade, M. Dulce Madeira, and A. Cardoso. "Cafeteria-diet effects on cognitive functions, anxiety, fear response and neurogenesis in the juvenile rat." *Neurobiology of Learning and Memory* 155 (2018): pp. 197–207.

Fonnebo, V. "Mortality in Norwegian Seventh-Day Adventists 1962–1986." *Journal of Clinical Epidemiology* 45, no. 2 (1992): pp. 157–167.

Fontana, F., K. Bourbeau, T. Moriarty, and M.P. da Silva. "The Relationship between Physical Activity, Sleep Quality, and Stress: A Study of Teachers during the COVID-19 Pandemic." *International Journal of Environmental Research and Public Health* 19, no. 23 (2022): pp. 15465.

Food systems and diets: Facing the challenges of the 21st century. Global Panel on Agriculture and Food Systems for Nutrition, 2016. http://glopan.org/sites/default/files/ForesightReport.pdf.

Fountain, John, Jasleen Kaur, and Sarah Lappin. *Physiology, Renin Angiotensin System.* Treasure Island, FL: StatPearls Publishing, 2023.

Fraser, G.E., and D.J. Shavlik. "Ten years of life: Is it a matter of choice?" *Archives of Internal Medicine* 161, no. 13 (2001): pp. 1645–1652.

Frates, B., J.P. Bonnet, R. Joseph, J.A. Peterson. *Lifestyle Medicine Handbook.* Monterey, CA: Healthy Learning, 2019.

Gardner, C.D., J.F. Trepanowski, L.C. Del Gobbo, M.E. Hauser, J. Rigdon, J.P.A. Ioannidis, et al. "Effect of Low-Fat vs Low-Carbohydrate Diet on 12-Month Weight Loss in Overweight Adults and the Association With Genotype Pattern or Insulin Secretion: The DIETFITS Randomized Clinical Trial." *JAMA* 319, no. 7 (2018): pp. 667–679.

Gearhardt, A.N., and A.G. DiFeliceantonio. "Highly processed foods can be considered addictive substances based on established scientific criteria." *Addiction* 118, no. 4 (2023): pp. 589–598.

Gebel, K., D. Ding, T. Chey, E. Stamatakis, W.J. Brown, and A.E. Bauman. "Effect of Moderate to Vigorous Physical Activity on All-Cause Mortality in Middle-aged and Older Australians." *JAMA Internal Medicine* 175, no. 6 (2015): pp. 970–977.

Geier, S.A. "Placebos in medicine." *The Lancet* 344, no. 8937 (1994): p. 1642.

Gentilcore, D., R. Chaikomin, K.L. Jones, A. Russo, C. Feinle-Bisset, J.M. Wishart, et al. "Effects of fat on gastric emptying of and the glycemic, insulin, and incretin responses to a carbohydrate meal in type 2 diabetes." *Journal of Clinical Endocrinology and Metabolism* 91, no. 6 (2006): pp. 2062–2067.

Gibson, H., N. Carroll, J.E. Clague, and R.H. Edwards. "Exercise performance and fatiguability in patients with chronic fatigue syndrome." *Journal of Neurology, Neurosurgery, and Psychiatry* 56, no. 9 (1993): pp. 993–998.

Goessl, V.C., J.E. Curtiss, and S.G. Hofmann. "The effect of heart rate variability biofeedback training on stress and anxiety: a meta-analysis." *Psychological Medicine* 47, no. 15 (2017): pp. 2578–2586.

Goldstein, J.L., and M.S. Brown. "A century of cholesterol and coronaries: from plaques to genes to statins." *Cell* 161, no. 1 (2015): pp. 161–172.

Gopinath, B., G. Liew, D. Tang, G. Burlutsky, V.M. Flood, and P. Mitchell. "Consumption of eggs and the 15-year incidence of age-related macular degeneration." *Clinical Nutrition* 39, no. 2 (2020): pp. 580–584.

Gotzsche, P.C., and P.K. Gotzsche. "Cognitive behavioural therapy halves the risk of repeated suicide attempts: systematic review." *Journal of the Royal Society of Medicine* 110, no. 10 (2017): pp. 404–410.

Greenberg, D., and J.V. St. Peter. "Sugars and Sweet Taste: Addictive or Rewarding?" *International Journal of Environmental Research and Public Health* 18, no. 18 (2021): p. 9791.

Grodin, E.N., E. Burnette, B. Towns, A. Venegas, and L.A. Ray. "Effect of alcohol, tobacco, and cannabis co-use on gray matter volume in heavy drinkers." *Psychology of Addictive Behaviors* 35, no. 6 (2021): pp. 760–768.

Grosso, G., A. Micek, J. Godos, S. Sciacca, A. Pajak, M.A. Martinez-Gonzalez, et al. "Coffee consumption and risk of all-cause, cardiovascular, and cancer mortality in smokers and non-smokers: a dose-response meta-analysis." *European Journal of Epidemiology* 31, no. 12 (2016): pp. 1191–1205.

Gualano, M.R., F. Bert, M. Martorana, G. Voglino, V. Andriolo, R. Thomas, et al. "The long-term effects of bibliotherapy in depression treatment: Systematic review of randomized clinical trials." *Clinical Psychology Review* 58 (2017): pp. 49–58.

Guarneiri, L.L., and J.A. Cooper. "Intake of Nuts or Nut Products Does Not Lead to Weight Gain, Independent of Dietary Substitution Instructions: A Systematic Review and Meta-Analysis of Randomized Trials." *Advances in Nutrition* 12, no. 2 (2021): pp. 384–401.

Guasch-Ferre, M., Y. Li, W.C. Willett, Q. Sun, L. Sampson, J. Salas-Salvado, et al. "Consumption of Olive Oil and Risk of Total and Cause-Specific

Mortality Among U.S. Adults." *Journal of the American College of Cardiology* 79, no. 2 (2022): pp. 101–112.

Guo, Q., A. Ye, N. Bellissimo, H. Singh, and D. Rousseau. "Modulating fat digestion through food structure design." *Progress in Lipid Research* 68 (2017): pp. 109–118.

Haap, M., J. Machann, C. von Friedeburg, F. Schick, N. Stefan, N.F. Schwenzer, et al. "Insulin sensitivity and liver fat: role of iron load." *Journal of Clinical Endocrinology and Metabolism* 96, no. 6 (2011): pp. E958–961.

Haines, M., D. Broom, J. Stephenson, and W. Gillibrand. "Influence of Sprint Duration during Minimal Volume Exercise on Aerobic Capacity and Affect." *International Journal of Sports Medicine* 42, no. 4 (2021): pp. 357–364.

Halberg, N., T. Khan, M.E. Trujillo, I. Wernstedt-Asterholm, A.D. Attie, S. Sherwani, et al. "Hypoxia-inducible factor 1alpha induces fibrosis and insulin resistance in white adipose tissue." Molecular and Cellular Biology 29, no. 16 (2009): pp. 4467–4483.

Hall, K.D., A. Ayuketah, R. Brychta, H. Cai, T. Cassimatis, K.Y. Chen, et al. "Ultra-Processed Diets Cause Excess Calorie Intake and Weight Gain: An Inpatient Randomized Controlled Trial of Ad Libitum Food Intake." *Cell Metabolism* 30, no. 1 (2019): p. 226.

Harris, T., E.S. Limb, F. Hosking, I. Carey, S. DeWilde, C. Furness, et al. "Effect of pedometer-based walking interventions on long-term health outcomes: Prospective 4-year follow-up of two randomised controlled trials using routine primary care data." *PLOS Medicine* 16, no. 6 (2019): e1002836.

"Heart Failure Diet: Foods To Eat and Avoid." Cleveland Clinic, May 1, 2023. https://my.clevelandclinic.org/health/articles/15426-sodium-controlled-diet.

Heissel, A., D. Heinen, L.L. Brokmeier, N. Skarabis, M. Kangas, D. Vancampfort, et al. "Exercise as medicine for depressive symptoms? A systematic review and meta-analysis with meta-regression." *British Journal of Sports Medicine* 57, no. 16 (2023): pp. 1049–1057.

"Herodotus on Cyrus' capture of Babylon." Livius. https://www.livius.org/sources/content/herodotus/cyrus-takes-babylon/ (last modified July 14, 2020).

Hickie, I.B., S.L. Naismith, R. Robillard, E.M. Scott, and D.F. Hermens. "Manipulating the sleep-wake cycle and circadian rhythms to improve clinical management of major depression." *BMC Medicine* 11, no. 79 (2013).

Ho, F.K., Z. Zhou, F. Petermann-Rocha, S. Para-Soto, J. Boonpor, P. Welsh, et al. "Association Between Device-Measured Physical Activity and Incident Heart Failure: A Prospective Cohort Study of 94 739 UK Biobank Participants." Circulation 146, no. 12 (2022): pp. 883–891.

Howarth, N.C., T.T. Huang, S.B. Roberts, B.H. Lin, and M.A. McCrory. "Eating patterns and dietary composition in relation to BMI in younger and older adults." *International Journal of Obesity* 31, no. 4 (2007): pp. 675–684.

Hua, N.W., R.A. Stoohs, and F.S. Facchini. "Low iron status and enhanced insulin sensitivity in lacto-ovo vegetarians." *British Journal of Nutrition* 86, no. 4 (2001): pp. 515–519.

Hur, J., F. Otegbeye, H.K. Joh, K. Nimptsch, K. Ng, S. Ogino, et al. "Sugar-sweetened beverage intake in adulthood and adolescence and risk of early-onset colorectal cancer among women." *Gut* 70, no. 12 (2021): pp. 2330–2336.

Hussain, M.Z., and A. Ahad. "Tablet colour in anxiety states." *British Medical Journal* 3, no. 5720 (1970): p. 466.

Hutton, T.M., S.T. Aaronson, L.L. Carpenter, K. Pages, W.S. West, C. Kraemer, et al. "The Anxiolytic and Antidepressant Effects of Transcranial Magnetic Stimulation in Patients With Anxious Depression." *Journal of Clinical Psychiatry* 84, no. 1 (2023): 22m14571.

Jacquart, J., C.D. Dutcher, S.Z. Freeman, A.T. Stein, M. Dinh, E. Carl, et al. "The effects of exercise on transdiagnostic treatment targets: A meta-analytic review." *Behaviour Research and Therapy* 115 (2019): pp. 19–37.

Jakobs, K., and C. Seez. "The Higgs Boson discovery." *Scholarpedia* 10, no. 9 (2015).

Jakubowicz, D., Z. Landau, S. Tsameret, J. Wainstein, I. Raz, B. Ahren, et al. "Reduction in Glycated Hemoglobin and Daily Insulin Dose Alongside Circadian Clock Upregulation in Patients With Type 2 Diabetes Consuming a Three-Meal Diet: A Randomized Clinical Trial." *Diabetes Care* 42, no. 12 (2019): pp. 2171–2180.

Jakubowicz, D., J. Wainstein, S. Tsameret, and Z. Landau. "Role of High Energy Breakfast 'Big Breakfast Diet' in Clock Gene Regulation of

Postprandial Hyperglycemia and Weight Loss in Type 2 Diabetes." *Nutrients* 13, no. 5 (2021): p. 1558.

James, K.A., J.I. Stromin, N. Steenkamp, and M.I. Combrinck. "Understanding the relationships between physiological and psychosocial stress, cortisol and cognition." *Frontiers in Endocrinology (Lausanne)* 14 (2023): 1085950.

Jenkins, A.J., J.D. Best, R.L. Klein, and T.J. Lyons. "'Lipoproteins, glycoxidation and diabetic angiopathy.'" *Diabetes/Metabolism Research and Reviews* 20, no. 5 (2004): pp. 349–368.

Jia, Y., D. Guo, L. Sun, M. Shi, K. Zhang, P. Yang, et al. "Self-Reported Daytime Napping, Daytime Sleepiness, and Other Sleep Phenotypes in the Development of Cardiometabolic Diseases: A Mendelian Randomization Study." *European Journal of Preventive Cardiology* 29, no. 15 (2022): pp. 1982–1991.

Johnson, A.R., M.D. Wilkerson, B.P. Sampey, M.A. Troester, D.N. Hayes, and L. Makowski. "Cafeteria diet-induced obesity causes oxidative damage in white adipose." *Biochemical and Biophysical Research Communications* 473, no. 2 (2016): pp. 545–50.

Jones, J.M. "CODEX-aligned dietary fiber definitions help to bridge the 'fiber gap.'" *Nutrition Journal* 13, no. 34 (2014).

Jones, S.E., J.M. Lane, A.R. Wood, V.T. van Hees, J. Tyrrell, R.N. Beaumont, et al. "Genome-wide association analyses of chronotype in 697,828 individuals provides insights into circadian rhythms." *Nature Communications* 10, no. 1 (2019): p. 343.

Juste, Y.R., S. Kaushik, M. Bourdenx, R. Aflakpui, S. Bandyopadhyay, F. Garcia, et al. "Reciprocal regulation of chaperone-mediated autophagy and the circadian clock." *Nature Cell Biology* 23, no. 12 (2021): pp. 1255–1270.

Kade, A.K., E.A. Chabanets, S.A. Zanin, and P.P. Polyakov. "Sick fat (adiposopathy) as the main contributor to metabolic syndrome." *Voprosy Pitaniia* 91, no. 1 (2022): pp. 27–36.

Kahleova, H., J.I. Lloren, A. Mashchak, M. Hill, and G.E. Fraser. "Meal Frequency and Timing Are Associated with Changes in Body Mass Index in Adventist Health Study 2." *Journal of Nutrition* 147, no. 9 (2017): pp. 1722–1728.

Kang, J., T. Jia, Z. Jiao, C. Shen, C. Xie, W. Cheng, et al. "Increased brain volume from higher cereal and lower coffee intake: shared genetic determinants and impacts on cognition and metabolism." *Cerebral Cortex* 32, no. 22 (2022): pp. 5163–5174.

Kaushik, S., Y.R. Juste, and A.M. Cuervo. "Circadian remodeling of the proteome by chaperone-mediated autophagy." *Autophagy* 18, no. 5 (2022): pp. 1205–1207.

Keast, R., A. Costanzo, and I. Hartley. "Macronutrient Sensing in the Oral Cavity and Gastrointestinal Tract: Alimentary Tastes." *Nutrients* 13, no. 2 (2021): p. 667.

Kelkar, P., and M.A. Ross. "Natural history of disease and placebo effect." *Perspectives in Biology and Medicine* 37, no. 2 (1994): pp. 244–246.

Kennedy, W.P. "The nocebo reaction." {*Medical World?*} 95 (1961): pp. 203–205.

Kessler, R.C., W.T. Chiu, O. Demler, K.R. Merikangas, and E.E. Walters. "Prevalence, severity, and comorbidity of 12-month DSM-IV disorders in the National Comorbidity Survey Replication." *Archives of General Psychiatry* 62, no. 6 (2005): pp. 617–627.

Khalighi Sikaroudi, M., S. Saraf-Bank, Z.S. Clayton, and S. Soltani. "A positive effect of egg consumption on macular pigment and healthy vision: a systematic review and meta-analysis of clinical trials." *Journal of the Science of Food and Agriculture* 101, no. 10 (2021): pp. 4003–4009.

Khan, A., J. Faucett, P. Lichtenberg, I. Kirsch, and W.A. Brown. "A systematic review of comparative efficacy of treatments and controls for depression." *PLOS One* 7, no. 7 (2012): e41778.

Kim, C., T. Okabe, M. Sakurai, K. Kanaya, K. Ishihara, T. Inoue, et al. "Gastric emptying of a carbohydrate-electrolyte solution in healthy volunteers depends on osmotically active particles." *Journal of Nippon Medical School* 80, no. 5 (2013): pp. 342–349.

Kirsch, I. "Placebo Effect in the Treatment of Depression and Anxiety." *Frontiers in Psychiatry* 10 (2019): p. 407.

Kleibeuker, J.H., H. Beekhuis, J.B. Jansen, D.A. Piers, and C.B. Lamers. "Cholecystokinin is a physiological hormonal mediator of fat-induced inhibition of gastric emptying in man." *European Journal of Clinical Investigation* 18, no. 2 (1988): pp. 173–177.

Koonin, E.V. "The Biological Big Bang model for the major transitions in evolution." *Biology Direct* 2, no. 21 (2007).

Koopman, K.E., M.W. Caan, A.J. Nederveen, A. Pels, M.T. Ackermans, E. Fliers, et al. "Hypercaloric diets with increased meal frequency, but not meal size, increase intrahepatic triglycerides: a randomized controlled trial." Hepatology 60, no. 2 (2014): pp. 545–553.

Koppes, Steve. "The Origin of Life on Earth, explained." *University of Chicago News*, September 19, 2022.

Krijnen-de Bruin, E., W. Scholten, A. Muntingh, O. Maarsingh, B. van Meijel, A. van Straten, et al. "Psychological interventions to prevent relapse in anxiety and depression: A systematic review and meta-analysis." *PLOS One* 17, no. 8 (2022): e0272200.

Kuo CL, Pilling LC, Kuchel GA, Ferrucci L, and D. Melzer. "Telomere length and aging-related outcomes in humans: A Mendelian randomization study in 261,000 older participants." *Aging Cell* 18, no. 6 (2019): e13017.

Lattimer, J.M., and M.D. Haub. "Effects of dietary fiber and its components on metabolic health." *Nutrients* 2, no. 12 (2010): pp. 1266–1289.

Leamy, A.K., C.M. Hasenour, R.A. Egnatchik, I.A. Trenary, C.H. Yao, G.J. Patti, et al. "Knockdown of triglyceride synthesis does not enhance palmitate lipotoxicity or prevent oleate-mediated rescue in rat hepatocytes." *Biochimica et Biophysica Acta* 1861, no. 9, pt A (2016): pp. 1005–1014.

Lee, D.C., X. Sui, E.G. Artero, I.M. Lee, T.S. Church, P.A. McAuley, et al. "Long-term effects of changes in cardiorespiratory fitness and body mass index on all-cause and cardiovascular disease mortality in men: the Aerobics Center Longitudinal Study." *Circulation* 124, no. 23 (2011): pp. 2483–2490.

Lee, K.H., H.J. Seong, G. Kim, G.H. Jeong, J.Y. Kim, H. Park, et al. "Consumption of Fish and omega-3 Fatty Acids and Cancer Risk: An Umbrella Review of Meta-Analyses of Observational Studies." *Advances in Nutrition* 11, no. 5 (2020): pp. 1134–1149.

Lee, P.H., Y.A. Feng, and J.W. Smoller. "Pleiotropy and Cross-Disorder Genetics Among Psychiatric Disorders." *Biological Psychiatry* 89, no. 1 (2021): pp. 20–31.

Legård, Grit, and Bente Pedersen. "Muscle as an Endocrine Organ." Chap. 13 in *Muscle and Exercise Physiology*. London: Elsevier Inc., 2019.

Leigh, S.J., M.D. Kendig, and M.J. Morris. "Palatable Western-style Cafeteria Diet as a Reliable Method for Modeling Diet-induced Obesity in Rodents." *Journal of Visualized Experiments* 153 (2019).

Levkovitz, Y., M. Isserles, F. Padberg, S.H. Lisanby, A. Bystritsky, G. Xia, et al. "Efficacy and safety of deep transcranial magnetic stimulation for major depression: a prospective multicenter randomized controlled trial." *World Psychiatry* 14, no. 1 (2015): pp. 64–73.

Lewinsohn, Peter, Ricardo Munoz, Mary Ann Youngren, and Antoinette Zeiss. *Control Your Depression.* Rev'd ed. New York: Simon & Schuster, 1992.

Lin, Y.S., J. Weibel, H.P. Landolt, F. Santini, C. Garbazza, J. Kistler, et al. "Time to Recover From Daily Caffeine Intake." *Frontiers in Nutrition* 8 (2021): 787225.

Lin, Y.S., J. Weibel, H.P. Landolt, F. Santini, M. Meyer, J. Brunmair, et al. "Daily Caffeine Intake Induces Concentration-Dependent Medial Temporal Plasticity in Humans: A Multimodal Double-Blind Randomized Controlled Trial." *Cerebral Cortex* 31, no. 6 (2021): pp. 3096–3106.

Lindeberg, S., P. Nilsson-Ehle, A. Terent, B. Vessby, and B. Schersten. "Cardiovascular risk factors in a Melanesian population apparently free from stroke and ischaemic heart disease: the Kitava study." *Journal of Internal Medicine* 236, no. 3 (1994): pp. 331–340.

Lipke, K., A. Kubis-Kubiak, and A. Piwowar. "Molecular Mechanism of Lipotoxicity as an Interesting Aspect in the Development of Pathological States-Current View of Knowledge." *Cells* 11, no. 5 (2022): p. 844.

Lown, B. "Verbal conditioning of angina pectoris during exercise testing." *American Journal of Cardiology* 40, no. 4 (1977): pp. 630–634.

Lunsford-Avery, J.R., M.M. Engelhard, A.M. Navar, and S.H. Kollins. "Validation of the Sleep Regularity Index in Older Adults and Associations with Cardiometabolic Risk." *Scientific Reports* 8, no.1 (2018): p. 14158.

Luo, X.D., J.S. Feng, Z. Yang, Q.T. Huang, J.D. Lin, B. Yang, et al. "High-dose omega-3 polyunsaturated fatty acid supplementation might be more superior than low-dose for major depressive disorder in early therapy period: a network meta-analysis." *BMC Psychiatry* 20, no. 1 (2020): p. 248.

Luparello, T.J., N. Leist, C.H. Lourie, and P. Sweet. "The interaction of psychologic stimuli and pharmacologic agents on airway reactivity i n asthmatic subjects." *Psychosomatic Medicine* 32, no. 5 (1970): pp. 509–513.

Luukkonen, P.K., S. Sadevirta, Y. Zhou, B. Kayser, A. Ali, L. Ahonen, et al. "Saturated Fat Is More Metabolically Harmful for the Human Liver Than Unsaturated Fat or Simple Sugars." *Diabetes Care* 41, no. 8 (2018): pp. 1732–1739.

Lyell, Charles. *Life, Letters and Journals of Sir Charles Lyell, Bart,* Vol. 1. Edited by Mrs. Lyell. London: John Murray, 1881.

Ma, D., S. Panda, and J.D. Lin. "Temporal orchestration of circadian autophagy rhythm by C/EBPβ." *The EMBO Journal* 30, no. 22 (2011): pp. 4642–4651.

Macchi, M.M., and J.N. Bruce. "Human pineal physiology and functional significance of melatonin." *Frontiers in Neuroendocrinology* 25, nos. 3, 4 (2004): pp. 177–195.

Macklis, R.M. "The great radium scandal." *Scientific American* 269, no. 2 (1993): pp 94–99.

Makarem, N., E.V. Bandera, Y. Lin, P.F. Jacques, R.B. Hayes, and N. Parekh. "Consumption of Sugars, Sugary Foods, and Sugary Beverages in Relation to Adiposity-Related Cancer Risk in the Framingham Offspring Cohort (1991–2013)." *Cancer Prevention Research* 11, no. 6 (2018): pp. 347–358.

Malik, M.. "Heart rate variability: standards of measurement, physiological interpretation and clinical use. Task Force of the European Society of Cardiology and the North American Society of Pacing and Electrophysiology." *Circulation* 93, no. 5 (1996): pp. 1043–1065.

Malik, V.S., and F.B. Hu. "The role of sugar-sweetened beverages in the global epidemics of obesity and chronic diseases." *Nature Reviews Endocrinology* 18, no. 4 (2022): pp. 205–218.

Mammen, G., and G. Faulkner. "Physical activity and the prevention of depression: a systematic review of prospective studies." *American Journal of Preventive Medicine* 45, no. 5 (2013): pp. 649–657.

Mandsager, K., S. Harb, P. Cremer, D. Phelan, S.E. Nissen, and W. Jaber. "Association of Cardiorespiratory Fitness With Long-term Mortality Among Adults Undergoing Exercise Treadmill Testing." *JAMA Network Open* 1, no. 6 (2018): e183605.

Marcell, T.J., S.A. Hawkins, R.A. Wiswell. "Leg strength declines with advancing age despite habitual endurance exercise in active older adults." *Journal of Strength and Conditioning Research* 28, no. 2 (2014): pp. 504–513.

Martchenko, A., S.E. Martchenko, A.D. Biancolin, and P.L. Brubaker. "Circadian Rhythms and the Gastrointestinal Tract: Relationship to Metabolism and Gut Hormones." *Endocrinology* 161, no. 12 (2020).

Martinez Steele, E., D. Raubenheimer, S.J. Simpson, L.G. Baraldi, and C.A. Monteiro. "Ultra-processed foods, protein leverage and energy intake in the USA." *Public Health Nutrition* 21, no. 1 (2018): pp. 114–124.

Martin-Soelch, C., A.F. Chevalley, G. Kunig, J. Missimer, S. Magyar, A. Mino, et al. "Changes in reward-induced brain activation in opiate addicts." *European Journal of Neuroscience* 14, no. 8 (2001): pp. 1360–1368.

Masana, M.F., J.M. Haro, A. Mariolis, S. Piscopo, G. Valacchi, V. Bountziouka, et al. "Mediterranean diet and depression among older individuals: The multinational MEDIS study." *Experimental Gerontology* 110 (2018): pp. 67–72.

Maslej, M.M., B.M. Bolker, M.J. Russell, K. Eaton, Z. Durisko, S.D. Hollon, et al. "The Mortality and Myocardial Effects of Antidepressants Are Moderated by Preexisting Cardiovascular Disease: A Meta-Analysis." *Psychotherapy and Psychosomatics* 86, no. 5 (2017): pp. 268–282.

Matochik, J.A., E.D. London, D.A. Eldreth, J.L. Cadet, and K.I. Bolla. "Frontal cortical tissue composition in abstinent cocaine abusers: a magnetic resonance imaging study." *NeuroImage* 19, no. 3 (2003): pp. 1095–1102.

McArthur, B.M., and R.D. Mattes. "Energy extraction from nuts: walnuts, almonds and pistachios." *British Journal of Nutrition* 123, no. 4 (2020): pp. 361–371.

McCormack, J., and C. Korownyk. "Effectiveness of antidepressants." *The BMJ* 360 (2018): k1073.

McCrory, M.A., and W.W. Campbell. "Effects of eating frequency, snacking, and breakfast skipping on energy regulation: symposium overview." *Journal of Nutrition* 141, no. 1 (2011): pp. 144–147.

McDonald, R.B., and J.J. Ramsey. "Honoring Clive McCay and 75 years of calorie restriction research." *The Journal of Nutrition* 140, no. 7 (2010): pp. 1205–1210.

McMahon, F.G. "Placebos in medicine." *The Lancet* 344, no. 8937 (1994): p. 1641.

Mekary, R.A., E. Giovannucci, L. Cahill, W.C. Willett, R.M. van Dam, and F.B. Hu. "Eating patterns and type 2 diabetes risk in older women: breakfast consumption and eating frequency." *American Journal of Clinical Nutrition* 98, no. 2 (2013): pp. 436–443.

Mekary, R.A., E. Giovannucci, W.C. Willett, R.M. van Dam, and F.B. Hu. "Eating patterns and type 2 diabetes risk in men: breakfast omission, eating frequency, and snacking." *American Journal of Clinical Nutrition* 95, no. 5 (2012): pp. 1182–1189.

Meng, L., W. Hou, J. Chui, R. Han, and A.W. Gelb. "Cardiac Output and Cerebral Blood Flow: The Integrated Regulation of Brain Perfusion in Adult Humans." *Anesthesiology* 123, no. 5 (2015): pp. 1198–1208.

Merakou, K., K. Tsoukas, G. Stavrinos, E. Amanaki, A. Daleziou, N. Kourmousi, et al. "The Effect of Progressive Muscle Relaxation on Emotional Competence: Depression-Anxiety-Stress, Sense of Coherence, Health-Related Quality of Life, and Well-Being of Unemployed People in Greece: An Intervention Study." *Explore: The Journal of Science & Healing* 15, no. 1 (2019): pp. 38–46.

Merriam-Webster's Dictionary, s.v. "vitalism," https://www.merriam-webster.com/dictionary/vitalism (accessed April 22, 2024).

Metcalfe, R.S., F. Koumanov, J.S. Ruffino, K.A. Stokes, G.D. Holman, D. Thompson, et al. "Physiological and molecular responses to an acute bout of reduced-exertion high-intensity interval training (REHIT)." *European Journal of Applied Physiology* 115, no. 11 (2015): pp. 2321–2334.

Metcalfe, R.S., and N.B.J. Vollaard. "Heterogeneity and incidence of non-response for changes in cardiorespiratory fitness following time-efficient sprint interval exercise training." *Applied Physiology, Nutrition, and Metabolism* 46, no. 7 (2021): pp. 735–742.

Miller, F.G. "The enduring legacy of sham-controlled trials of internal mammary artery ligation." *Progress in Cardiovascular Diseases* 55, no. 3 (2012): pp. 246–250.

Miquel-Kergoat, S., V. Azais-Braesco, B. Burton-Freeman, and M.M. Hetherington. "Effects of chewing on appetite, food intake and gut hormones: A systematic review and meta-analysis." *Physiology & Behavior* 151 (2015): pp. 88–96.

Moncrieff, J. "What does the latest meta-analysis really tell us about antidepressants?" *Epidemiology and Psychiatric Sciences* 27, no. 5 (2018): pp. 430–432.

Monteiro, C.A., G. Cannon, J.C. Moubarac, R.B. Levy, M.L.C. Louzada, and P.C. Jaime. "The UN Decade of Nutrition, the NOVA food classification and the trouble with ultra-processing." *Public Health Nutrition* 21, no. 1 (2018): pp. 5–17.

Moor, Fred, Stella Peterson, Ethel Manwell, Mary Noble, and Gertrude Muench. *Manual of Hydrotherapy and Massage.* Mountain View, CA: Pacific Press Publishing Association, 1964.

Morey, J.N., I.A. Boggero, A.B. Scott, and S.C. Segerstrom. "Current Directions in Stress and Human Immune Function." *Current Opinion in Psychology* 5 (2015): pp. 13–17.

Mozaffarian, D., T. Hao, E.B. Rimm, W.C. Willett, and F.B. Hu. "Changes in diet and lifestyle and long-term weight gain in women and men." *New England Journal of Medicine* 364, no. 25 (2011): pp. 2392–2404.

Mozaffarian, D., M.B. Katan, A. Ascherio, M.J. Stampfer, W.C. Willett. "Trans fatty acids and cardiovascular disease." *The New England Journal of Medicine* 354, no. 15 (2006): pp. 1601–1613.

Mozaffarian, R.S., R.M. Lee, M.A. Kennedy, D.S. Ludwig, D. Mozaffarian, and S.L. Gortmaker. "Identifying whole grain foods: a comparison of different approaches for selecting more healthful whole grain products." *Public Health Nutrition* 16, no. 12 (2013): pp. 2255–2264.

Munoz, R.F., W.R. Beardslee, and Y. Leykin. "Major depression can be prevented." *American Psychologist* 67, no. 4 (2012): pp. 285–295.

Myers, J., M. Prakash, V. Froelicher, D. Do, S. Partington, and J.E. Atwood. "Exercise capacity and mortality among men referred for exercise testing." *New England Journal of Medicine* 346, no. 11 (2002): pp. 793–801.

N. C. D. Risk Factor Collaboration. "Worldwide trends in body-mass index, underweight, overweight, and obesity from 1975 to 2016: a pooled analysis of 2416 population-based measurement studies in 128.9 million children, adolescents, and adults." *The Lancet* 390, no. 10113 (2017): pp. 2627–2642.

Nagao, K., and T. Yanagita. "Medium-chain fatty acids: functional lipids for the prevention and treatment of the metabolic syndrome." *Pharmacological Research* 61, no. 3 (2010): pp. 208–212.

Nakao, K., A. Ro, and K. Kibayashi. "Evaluation of the morphological changes of gastric mucosa induced by a low concentration of acetic acid using a rat model." *Journal of Forensic and Legal Medicine* 22 (2014): pp. 99–106.

Nalcakan, G.R., P. Songsorn, B.L. Fitzpatrick, Y. Yuzbasioglu, N.E. Brick, R.S. Metcalfe, et al. "Decreasing sprint duration from 20 to 10 s during reduced-exertion high-intensity interval training (REHIT) attenuates the increase in maximal aerobic capacity but has no effect on affective and perceptual responses." *Applied Physiology, Nutrition, and Metabolism* 43, no. 4 (2018): pp. 338–344.

Natalucci, G., S. Riedl, A. Gleiss, T. Zidek, and H. Frisch. "Spontaneous 24-h ghrelin secretion pattern in fasting subjects: maintenance of a meal-related pattern." *European Journal of Endocrinology* 152, no. 6 (2005): pp. 845–850.

National Research Council and Institute of Medicine. *Preventing Mental, Emotional, and Behavioral Disorders Among Young People: Progress and Possibilities*. Washington, D.C.: The National Academies Press, 2009.

The National Weight Control Registry. http://www.nwcr.ws/ (accessed June 27, 2022).

Neuhouser, M.L., B.C. Wertheim, M.M. Perrigue, M. Hingle, L.F. Tinker, M. Shikany, et al. "Associations of Number of Daily Eating Occasions with Type 2 Diabetes Risk in the Women's Health Initiative Dietary Modification Trial." *Current Developments in Nutrition* 4, no. 8 (2020): nzaa126.

Newby, J.M., C. Twomey, S.S. Yuan Li, and G. Andrews. "Transdiagnostic computerised cognitive behavioural therapy for depression and anxiety: A systematic review and meta-analysis." *Journal of Affective Disorders* 199 (2016): pp. 30–41.

Newman, A.B., V. Kupelian, M. Visser, E.M. Simonsick, B.H. Goodpaster, S.B. Kritchevsky, et al. "Strength, but not muscle mass, is associated with mortality in the health, aging and body composition study cohort." *Journals of Gerontology Series A: Biological Sciences and Medical Sciences* 61, no. 1 (2006): pp. 72–77.

NHLBI. "What is Metabolic Syndrome?" National Heart, Lung, and Blood Institute, https://www.nhlbi.nih.gov/health-topics/metabolic-syndrome (accessed April 22, 2024).

Nichol, Francis D. *Why I Believe in Mrs. E. G. White.* Silver Spring, MD: The White Estate, Inc.; 1964.

NIMH. "What is Depression?" National Institute of Mental Health https://www.nimh.nih.gov/health/publications/depression (accessed April 22, 2024).

Nolan, C.J., and C.Z. Larter. "Lipotoxicity: why do saturated fatty acids cause and monounsaturates protect against it?" *Journal of Gastroenterology and Hepatology* 24, no. 5 (2009): pp. 703–706.

Normand, M., C. Ritz, D. Mela, and A. Raben. "Low-energy sweeteners and body weight: a citation network analysis." *BMJ Nutrition, Prevention & Health* 4, no. 1 (2021): pp. 319–332.

"Obesity and overweight." World Health Organization. https://www.who.int/news-room/fact-sheets/detail/obesity-and-overweight, June 9, 2021.

Ogawa, Y., K. Imajo, Y. Honda, T. Kessoku, W. Tomeno, S. Kato, et al. "Palmitate-induced lipotoxicity is crucial for the pathogenesis of nonalcoholic fatty liver disease in cooperation with gut-derived endotoxin." *Scientific Reports* 8, no. 1 (2018): p. 11365.

Ohkawara K, M.A. Cornier, W.M. Kohrt, and E.L. Melanson. "Effects of increased meal frequency on fat oxidation and perceived hunger." *Obesity* 21, no. 2 (2013): pp. 336–343.

Ohkuma, T., Y. Hirakawa, U. Nakamura, Y. Kiyohara, T. Kitazono, and T. Ninomiya. "Association between eating rate and obesity: a systematic review and meta-analysis." *International Journal of Obesity* 39, no. 11 (2015): pp. 1589–1596.

Okabe, S., and K. Amagase. "An overview of acetic acid ulcer models-- the history and state of the art of peptic ulcer research." *Biological and Pharmaceutical Bulletin* 28, no. 8 (2005): pp. 1321–1341.

Oliveira, E.R., N.V. Cade, A.P. Velten, G.A. Silva, and E. Faerstein. "Comparative study of cardiovascular and cancer mortality of Adventists and non-Adventists from Espirito Santo State, in the period from 2003 to 2009." *Brazilian Journal of Epidemiology* 19, no. 1 (2016): pp. 112–121.

Orlich, M.J., J. Sabate, A. Mashchak, U. Fresan, K. Jaceldo-Siegl, F. Miles, et al. "Ultra-processed food intake and animal-based food intake and mortality in the Adventist health study-2." *American Journal of Clinical Nutrition* 115, no. 6 (2022): 1589–1601.

Orlich, M.J., P.N. Singh, J. Sabate, K. Jaceldo-Siegl, J. Fan, S. Knutsen S, et al. "Vegetarian dietary patterns and mortality in Adventist Health Study 2." JAMA Internal Medicine 173, no. 13 (2013): pp. 1230–1238.

Oshima, M., S. Pechberty, L. Bellini, S.O. Gopel, M. Campana, C. Rouch, et al. "Stearoyl CoA desaturase is a gatekeeper that protects human beta cells against lipotoxicity and maintains their identity." Diabetologia 63, no. 2 (2020): pp. 395–409.

O'Sullivan, T.A., K. Hafekost, F. Mitrou, and D. Lawrence. "Food sources of saturated fat and the association with mortality: a meta-analysis." American Journal of Public Health 103, no. 9 (2013): pp. e31–42.

Pacha, J., and A. Sumova. "Circadian regulation of epithelial functions in the intestine." Acta Physiologica 208, no. 1 (2013): pp. 11–24.

Parry, S.A., F. Rosqvist, F.E. Mozes, T. Cornfield, M. Hutchinson, M.E. Piche, et al. "Intrahepatic Fat and Postprandial Glycemia Increase After Consumption of a Diet Enriched in Saturated Fat Compared With Free Sugars." Diabetes Care 43, no. 5 (2020): pp. 1134–1141.

Patel, A.V., J.M. Hodge, E. Rees-Punia, L.R. Teras, P.T. Campbell, and S.M. Gapstur. "Relationship Between Muscle-Strengthening Activity and Cause-Specific Mortality in a Large US Cohort." Preventing Chronic Disease 17 (2020): p. E78.

Patton, A.P., and M.H. Hastings. "The suprachiasmatic nucleus." Current Biology 28, n. 15 (2018): pp. R816–R822.

Peng, Z., P. Wu, J. Wang, D. Dupont, O. Menard, R. Jeantet, et al. "Achieving realistic gastric emptying curve in an advanced dynamic in vitro human digestion system: experiences with cheese—a difficult to empty material." Food & Function 12, no. 9 (2021): pp. 3965–3977.

Pennington, J.A.T. Food Values of Portions Commonly Used. 15th ed. New York: Harper Collins, 1989.

Perez-Cornago, A., A. Sanchez-Villegas, M. Bes-Rastrollo, A. Gea, P. Molero, F. Lahortiga-Ramos, et al. "Relationship between adherence to Dietary Approaches to Stop Hypertension (DASH) diet indices and incidence of depression during up to 8 years of follow-up." Public Health Nutrition 20, no. 13 (2017): pp. 2383–2392.

Peruri, A., A. Morgan, A. D'Souza, B. Mellon, C.W. Hung, G. Kayal, et al. "Pineal Gland from the Cell Culture to Animal Models: A Review." Life 12, no. 7 (2022).

Peters, J.C. "Dietary fat and body weight control." *Lipids* 38, no. 2 (2003): pp. 123–127.

Pettersson, E., H. Larsson, and P. Lichtenstein. "Common psychiatric disorders share the same genetic origin: a multivariate sibling study of the Swedish population." *Molecular Psychiatry* 21, no. 5 (2016): pp. 717–721.

Phillips, A.J.K, W.M. Clerx, C.S. O'Brien, A. Sano, L.K. Barger, R.W. Picard, et al. "Irregular sleep/wake patterns are associated with poorer academic performance and delayed circadian and sleep/wake timing." *Scientific Reports* 7, no. 1 (2017): p. 3216.

Piliavin, J.A., and E. Siegl. "Health benefits of volunteering in the Wisconsin longitudinal study." *Journal of Health and Social Behavior* 48, no. 4 (2007): pp. 450–464.

Plana-Ripoll O, Pedersen CB, Holtz Y, Benros ME, Dalsgaard S, de Jonge P, et al. "Exploring Comorbidity Within Mental Disorders Among a Danish National Population." *JAMA Psychiatry* 76, no. 3 (2019): pp. 259–270.

Popper, Karl. *Conjectures and Refutations*. San Francisco: Harper & Row, 1968.

Poppitt, S.D., and A.M. Prentice. "Energy density and its role in the control of food intake: evidence from metabolic and community studies." *Appetite* 26, no. 2 (1996): pp. 153–174.

Ramsden, C.E., K.R. Faurot, P. Carrera-Bastos, L. Cordain, M. De Lorgeril, and L.S. Sperling. "Dietary fat quality and coronary heart disease prevention: a unified theory based on evolutionary, historical, global, and modern perspectives." *Current Treatment Options in Cardiovascular Medicine* 11, no. 4 (2009): pp. 289–301.

Ravnskov, U., A. Alabdulgader, M. de Lorgeril, D.M. Diamond, R. Hama, T. Hamazaki, et al. "The new European guidelines for prevention of cardiovascular disease are misleading." *Expert Review of Clinical Pharmacology* 13, no. 12 (2020): pp. 1289–1294.

Ravnskov, U., M. de Lorgeril, D.M. Diamond, R. Hama, T. Hamazaki, B. Hammarskjold, et al. "LDL-C does not cause cardiovascular disease: a comprehensive review of the current literature." *Expert Review of Clinical Pharmacology* 11, no. 10 (2018): pp. 959–970.

Raynor, H.A., R.W. Jeffery, S. Phelan, J.O. Hill, and R.R. Wing. "Amount of food group variety consumed in the diet and long-term weight loss maintenance." *Obesity Research* 13, no. 5 (2005): pp. 883–890.

Reynolds, S.S., and C. Sova. "Memes and Poetry: A Descriptive Analysis on Creative Arts Therapy to Reduce Health Care Worker Burnout." *Journal of Nursing Care Quality* 37, no. 3 (2022): pp. 245–248.

Riad, M., M. Mogos, D. Thangathurai, and P.D. Lumb. "Steroids." *Current Opinion in Critical Care* 8, no. 4 (2002): pp. 281–284.

Richter, J., N. Herzog, S. Janka, T. Baumann, A. Kistenmacher, and K.M. Oltmanns. "Twice as High Diet-Induced Thermogenesis After Breakfast vs Dinner On High-Calorie as Well as Low-Calorie Meals." *Journal of Clinical Endocrinology and Metabolism* 105, no. 3 (2020): pp. e211–e221.

Robinson, E., E. Almiron-Roig, F. Rutters, C. de Graaf, C.G. Forde, C. Tudur Smith, et al. "A systematic review and meta-analysis examining the effect of eating rate on energy intake and hunger." *American Journal of Clinical Nutrition* 100, no. 1 (2014): pp. 123–151.

Rodak, K., I. Kokot, and E.M. Kratz. "Caffeine as a Factor Influencing the Functioning of the Human Body—Friend or Foe?" *Nutrients* 13, no. 9 (2021): p. 3088.

Rolls, B.J. "Plenary Lecture 1: Dietary strategies for the prevention and treatment of obesity." *Proceedings of the Nutrition Society* 69, no. 1 (2010): pp. 70–79.

Rolls, Barbara. *The Ultimate Volumetrics Diet*. New York: HarperCollins Publishers, 2013.

Ronis, M.J., J.N. Baumgardner, N. Sharma, J. Vantrease, M. Ferguson, Y. Tong, et al. "Medium chain triglycerides dose-dependently prevent liver pathology in a rat model of non-alcoholic fatty liver disease." *Experimental Biology and Medicine* 238, no. 2 (2013): pp. 151–162.

Rosqvist, F., D. Iggman, J. Kullberg, J. Cedernaes, H.E. Johansson, A. Larsson, et al. "Overfeeding polyunsaturated and saturated fat causes distinct effects on liver and visceral fat accumulation in humans." *Diabetes* 63, no. 7 (2014): pp. 2356–2368.

Roth, A.A. "'Flat gaps' in sedimentary rock layers challenge long geologic ages." *Journal of Creation* 23, no. 2 (2009): pp. 76–81.

Roth, Ariel. "Was There A Great Genesis Flood?" Geoscience Research Institute, https://www.grisda.org/was-there-a-great-genesis-flood-1, July 8, 2014.

Roy, A.L., and R.S. Conroy. "Toward mapping the human body at a cellular resolution." *Molecular Biology of the Cell* 29, no. 15 (2018): pp. 1779–1785.

Ruffino, J.S., P. Songsorn, M. Haggett, D. Edmonds, A.M. Robinson, D. Thompson, et al. "A comparison of the health benefits of reduced-exertion high-intensity interval training (REHIT) and moderate-intensity walking in type 2 diabetes patients." *Applied Physiology, Nutrition, and Metabolism* 42, no. 2 (2017): pp. 202–208.

Rynders, C.A., E.A Thomas, A. Zaman, Z. Pan, V.A. Catenacci, and E.L. Melanson. "Effectiveness of Intermittent Fasting and Time-Restricted Feeding Compared to Continuous Energy Restriction for Weight Loss." *Nutrients* 11, no. 10 (2019): p. 2442.

Sabate, J., N.M. Burkholder-Cooley, G. Segovia-Siapco, K. Oda, B. Wells, M.J. Orlich, et al. "Unscrambling the relations of egg and meat consumption with type 2 diabetes risk." *American Journal of Clinical Nutrition* 108, no. 5 (2018): pp. 1121–1128.

Sacks, F.M., A.H. Lichtenstein, J.H.Y. Wu, L.J. Appel, M.A. Creager, P.M. Kris-Etherton, et al. "Dietary Fats and Cardiovascular Disease: A Presidential Advisory From the American Heart Association." *Circulation* 136, no. 3 (2017): pp. e1–e23.

Sacks, F.M., L.P. Svetkey, W.M. Vollmer, L.J. Appel, G.A. Bray, D. Harsha, et al. "Effects on blood pressure of reduced dietary sodium and the Dietary Approaches to Stop Hypertension (DASH) diet. DASH-Sodium Collaborative Research Group." *New England Journal of Medicine* 344, no. 1 (2001): pp. 3–10.

Saha, S., D.P. Panigrahi, S. Patil, and S.K. Bhutia. "Autophagy in health and disease: A comprehensive review." *Biomedicine & Pharmacotherapy* 104, no. 2 (2018): pp. 485–495.

Salleh, M.R. "Life event, stress and illness." *Malaysian Journal of Medical Sciences* 15, no. 4 (2008): pp. 9–18.

Sallis, R.E., and L.W. Buckalew. "Relation of capsule color and perceived potency." *Perceptual and Motor Skills* 58, no. 3 (1984): pp. 897–898.

Sampey, B.P., A.M. Vanhoose, H.M. Winfield, A.J. Freemerman, M.J. Muehlbauer, P.T. Fueger, et al. "Cafeteria diet is a robust model of human metabolic syndrome with liver and adipose inflammation: comparison to high-fat diet." *Obesity* 19, no. 6 (2011): pp. 1109–1117.

Sayers, R.R. "Major Studies of Fatigue." *War Medicine* 2, no. 5 (1942): pp. 786–823.

Schaefer, J.D., A. Caspi, D.W. Belsky, H. Harrington, R. Houts, L.J. Horwood, et al. "Enduring mental health: Prevalence and prediction." *Journal of Abnormal Psychology* 126, no. 2 (2017): pp. 212–224.

Schapira, K., H.A. McClelland, N.R. Griffiths, and D.J. Newell. "Study on the effects of tablet colour in the treatment of anxiety states." *British Medical Journal* 1, no. 5707 (1970): pp. 446–449.

Schlechta Portella, C.F., R. Ghelman, V. Abdala, M.C. Schveitzer, and R.F. Afonso. "Meditation: Evidence Map of Systematic Reviews." *Frontiers in Public Health* 9 (2021): 742715.

Schoenfeld, B.J., B. Contreras, J. Krieger, J. Grgic, K. Delcastillo, R. Belliard, et al. "Resistance Training Volume Enhances Muscle Hypertrophy but Not Strength in Trained Men." *Medicine & Science in Sports & Exercise* 51, no. 1 (2019): pp. 94–103.

Schonfeld, P., and L. Wojtczak. "Short- and medium-chain fatty acids in energy metabolism: the cellular perspective." *Journal of Lipid Research* 57, no. 6 (2016): pp. 943–954.

Schweiger, A., and A. Parducci. "Nocebo: the psychologic induction of pain." *Pavlovian Journal of Biological Science* 16, no. 3 (1981): pp. 140–143.

Science and Creationism: A View from the National Academy of Sciences. 2nd ed. Washington, D.C.: The National Academies Press, 1999.

Segers, A., and I. Depoortere. "Circadian clocks in the digestive system." *Nature Reviews Gastroenterology & Hepatology* 18, no. 4 (2021): pp. 239–251.

Seguin, Rebecca, Jacqueline Epping, David Buchner, Rina Bloch, and Miriam Nelson. *Growing Stronger: Strength Training for Older Adults.* Washington, D.C.: U.S. Department of Health, 2002.

Seidelmann, S.B., B. Claggett, S. Cheng, M. Henglin, A. Shah, L.M. Steffen, et al. "Dietary carbohydrate intake and mortality: a prospective cohort study and meta-analysis." *Lancet Public Health* 3, no. 9 (2018): pp. e419–e428.

Shapiro, A.P., T. Myers, M.F. Reiser, and E.B. Ferris Jr. "Comparison of blood pressure response to veriloid and to the doctor." *Psychosomatic Medicine* 16, no. 6 (1954): pp. 478–488.

Sharpe, M., T. Chalder, and P.D. White. "Evidence-Based Care for People with Chronic Fatigue Syndrome and Myalgic Encephalomyelitis." *Journal of General Internal Medicine* 37, no. 2 (2022): pp. 449–452.

Shen, H., K. Eguchi, N. Kono, K. Fujiu, S. Matsumoto, M. Shibata, et al. "Saturated fatty acid palmitate aggravates neointima formation by promoting smooth muscle phenotypic modulation." Arteriosclerosis, Thrombosis, and Vascular Biology 33, no. 11 (2013): pp. 2596–2607.

Singh, B., T. Olds, R. Curtis, D. Dumuid, R. Virgara, A. Watson, et al. "Effectiveness of physical activity interventions for improving depression, anxiety and distress: an overview of systematic reviews." *British Journal of Sports Medicine* 57, no. 18 (2023): pp. 1203–1209.

Sisto, S.A., J. LaManca, D.L. Cordero, M.T. Bergen, S.P. Ellis, S. Drastal, et al. "Metabolic and cardiovascular effects of a progressive exercise test in patients with chronic fatigue syndrome." *American Journal of Medicine* 100, no. 6 (1996): pp. 634–640.

Slyper, A. "Oral Processing, Satiation and Obesity: Overview and Hypotheses." *Diabetes, Metabolic Syndrome and Obesity* 14 (2021): pp. 3399–3415.

Smith, N.M., M.R. Floyd, F. Scogin, and C.S. Jamison. "Three-year follow-up of bibliotherapy for depression." *Journal of Consulting and Clinical Psychology* 65, no. 2 (1997): pp. 324–327.

Smoller, J.W. "Disorders and borders: psychiatric genetics and nosology." *American Journal of Medical Genetics Part B: Neuropsychiatric Genetics* 162B, no. 7 (2013): pp. 559–578.

Snel, M., J.T. Jonker, J. Schoones, H. Lamb, A. de Roos, H. Pijl, et al. "Ectopic fat and insulin resistance: pathophysiology and effect of diet and lifestyle interventions." *International Journal of Endocrinology* 2012 (2012): p. 983814.

Son, H.K., W.Y. So, and M. Kim. "Effects of Aromatherapy Combined with Music Therapy on Anxiety, Stress, and Fundamental Nursing Skills in Nursing Students: A Randomized Controlled Trial." *International Journal of Environmental Research and Public Health* 16, no. 21 (2019): p. 4185.

Songsorn, P., A. Lambeth-Mansell, J.L. Mair, M. Haggett, B.L. Fitzpatrick, J. Ruffino, et al. Exercise training comprising of single 20-s cycle sprints does not provide a sufficient stimulus for improving maximal aerobic capacity in sedentary individuals." *European Journal of Applied Physiology* 116, no. 8 (2016): pp. 1511–1517.

Spigoni, V., F. Fantuzzi, A. Fontana, M. Cito, E. Derlindati, I. Zavaroni, et al. "Stearic acid at physiologic concentrations induces in vitro lipotoxicity in circulating angiogenic cells." *Atherosclerosis* 265, (2017): pp. 162–171.

Stamatikos, A.D., and C.M. Paton. "Role of stearoyl-CoA desaturase-1 in skeletal muscle function and metabolism." *American Journal of Physiology-Endocrinology and Metabolism* 305, no. 7 (2013): pp. E767–775.

Stanhope, J.M., and I.A. Prior. "The Tokelau Island migrant study: prevalence of various conditions before migration." *International Journal of Epidemiology* 5, no. 3 (1976): pp. 259–266.

Stanhope, J.M., V.M. Sampson, I.A. Prior. "The Tokelau Island Migrant Study: serum lipid concentration in two environments." *Journal of Chronic Diseases* 34, nos. 2, 3 (1981): pp. 45–55.

Sternbach, R.A. "The Effects of Instructional Sets on Autonomic Responsivity." *Psychophysiology* 1, no. 1 (1964): pp. 67–72.

Stice, E., P. Rohde, J.M. Gau, and E. Wade. "Efficacy trial of a brief cognitive-behavioral depression prevention program for high-risk adolescents: effects at 1- and 2-year follow-up." *Journal of Consulting and Clinical Psychology* 78, no. 6 (2010): pp. 856–867.

Stickel, F., and H.K. Seitz. "The efficacy and safety of comfrey. *Public Health Nutrition* 3, no. 4A (2000): pp. 501–508.

Straus, J.L., and S. von Ammon Cavanaugh. "Placebo effects. Issues for clinical practice in psychiatry and medicine." *Psychosomatics* 37, no. 4 (1996): pp. 315–326.

Stringham, J.M., E.J. Johnson, and B.R. Hammond. "Lutein across the Lifespan: From Childhood Cognitive Performance to the Aging Eye and Brain." Curr Dev Nutr 3, no. 7 (2019): nzz066.

Su, T.P., M.H. Chen, and P.C. Tu. "Using big data of genetics, health claims, and brain imaging to challenge the categorical classification in mental illness." *Journal of the Chinese Medical Association* 85, no. 2 (2022): pp. 139–144.

Sulc, J., N. Mounier, F. Gunther, T. Winkler, A.R. Wood, T.M. Frayling, et al. "Quantification of the overall contribution of gene-environment interaction for obesity-related traits." *Nature Communications* 11, no. 1 (2020): p. 1385.

Sutton, E.F., R. Beyl, K.S. Early, W.T. Cefalu, E. Ravussin, and C.M. Peterson. "Early Time-Restricted Feeding Improves Insulin Sensitivity, Blood Pressure, and Oxidative Stress Even without Weight Loss in Men with Prediabetes." *Cell Metabolism* 27, no. 6 (2018): pp. 1212–1221.e3.

Swinburn, B.A., G. Sacks, K.D. Hall, K. McPherson, D.T. Finegood, M.L. Moodie, et al. "The global obesity pandemic: shaped by global drivers and local environments." *The Lancet* 378, no. 9793 (2011): pp. 804–814.

Swithers, S.E. "Not-so-healthy sugar substitutes?" *Current Opinion in Behavioral Sciences* 9 (2016): pp. 106–110.

Taghizadeh, N., A. Eslaminejad, and M.R. Raoufy. "Protective effect of heart rate variability biofeedback on stress-induced lung function impairment in asthma." *Respiratory Physiology & Neurobiology* 262 (2019): pp. 49–56.

Takahashi, Y., D.M. Kipnis, and W.H. Daughaday. "Growth hormone secretion during sleep." *Journal of Clinical Investigation* 47, no. 9 (1968): pp. 2079–2090.

Takeda, Y., K. Ishibashi, Y. Kuroda, and G.I. Atsumi. "Exposure to Stearate Activates the IRE1alpha/XBP-1 Pathway in 3T3-L1 Adipocytes." Biological and Pharmaceutical Bulletin 44, no. 11 (2021): pp. 1752–1758.

Tappy, L., and K.A. Le. "Metabolic effects of fructose and the worldwide increase in obesity." *Physiological Reviews* 90, no. 1 (2010): pp. 23–46.

Taylor R. "Pathogenesis of type 2 diabetes: tracing the reverse route from cure to cause." *Diabetologia* 51, no. 10 (2008): pp. 1781–1789.

Taylor, J.J., C. Lin, D. Talmasov, M.A. Ferguson, F. Schaper, J. Jiang, et al. "A transdiagnostic network for psychiatric illness derived from atrophy and lesions." *Nature Human Behaviour* 7, no. 3 (2023): pp. 420–429.

Temple, N.J. "Fat, Sugar, Whole Grains and Heart Disease: 50 Years of Confusion." *Nutrients* 10, no. 1 (2018): p. 39.

Thomas, G., P. Songsorn, A. Gorman, B. Brackenridge, T. Cullen, B. Fitzpatrick, et al. "Reducing training frequency from 3 or 4 sessions/week to 2 sessions/week does not attenuate improvements in maximal aerobic capacity with reduced-exertion high-intensity interval training (REHIT)." *Applied Physiology, Nutrition, and Metabolism* 45, no. 6 (2020): pp. 583–685.

Thomas, K.B. "General practice consultations: is there any point in being positive?" *British Medical Journal (Clinical Research Edition)* 294, no. 6581 (1987): pp. 1200–1202.

Thompson, P.M., K.M. Hayashi, S.L. Simon, J.A. Geaga, M.S. Hong, Y. Sui, et al. "Structural abnormalities in the brains of human subjects who use methamphetamine." *Journal of Neuroscience* 24, no. 26 (2004): pp. 6028–6036.

"Tips for Better Sleep." Centers for Disease Control and Prevention https://www.cdc.gov/sleep/aboutsleep/sleep_hygiene.html (accessed April 22, 2024).

Toledo, F.G.S., D.L. Johannsen, J.D. Covington, S. Bajpeyi, B. Goodpaster, K.E. Conley, et al. "Impact of prolonged overfeeding on skeletal muscle mitochondria in healthy individuals." *Diabetologia* 61, no. 2 (2018): pp. 466–475.

Toussaint, L., Q.A. Nguyen, C. Roettger, K. Dixon, M. Offenbacher, N. Kohls, et al. "Effectiveness of Progressive Muscle Relaxation, Deep Breathing, and Guided Imagery in Promoting Psychological and Physiological States of Relaxation." *Evidence-Based Complementary and Alternative Medicine* 2021 (2021): 5924040.

"Treatment of ME/CFS." Centers for Disease Control and Prevention. https://www.cdc.gov/me-cfs/treatment/index.html (last reviewed January 28, 2021).

Tudor Hart, J., and P. Dieppe. "Caring effects." *The Lancet* 347, no. 9015 (1996): pp. 1606–1608.

Tudor-Locke, C., J. Mora-Gonzalez, S.W. Ducharme, E.J. Aguiar, J.M. Schuna Jr., T.V. Barreira, et al. "Walking cadence (steps/min) and intensity in 61-85-year-old adults: the CADENCE-Adults study." *International Journal of Behavioral Nutrition* Act 18, no. 1 (2021): p. 129.

Turner, J.A., R.A. Deyo, J.D. Loeser, M. Von Korff, and W.E. Fordyce. "The importance of placebo effects in pain treatment and research." *JAMA* 271, no. 20 (1994): pp. 1609–1614.

U.S. Department of Agriculture and U.S. Department of Health and Human Services. *Dietary Guidelines for Americans, 2020–2025.* 9th ed. 2020.

U.S. Department of Health and Human Services. *Physical Activity Guidelines for Americans.* 2nd ed. Washington, D.C: U.S. Department of Health and Human Services, 2018.

Ulgherait, M., A.M. Midoun, S.J. Park, J.A. Gatto, S.J. Tener, J. Siewert, et al. "Circadian autophagy drives iTRF-mediated longevity." *Nature* 598, no. 7880 (2021): pp. 353–358.

van der Zwan, J.E., W. de Vente, A.C. Huizink, S.M. Bogels, and E.I. de Bruin. "Physical activity, mindfulness meditation, or heart rate variability biofeedback for stress reduction: a randomized controlled trial." *Applied Psychophysiology and Biofeedback* 40, no. 4 (2015): pp. 257–268.

Vanbuskirk, K.A., and M.N. Potenza. "The Treatment of Obesity and Its Co-occurrence with Substance Use Disorders." *Journal of Addiction Medicine* 4, no. 1 (2010): pp. 1–10.

Vera, B., H.S. Dashti, P. Gomez-Abellan, A.M. Hernandez-Martinez, A. Esteban, F. Scheer, et al. "Modifiable lifestyle behaviors, but not a genetic risk score, associate with metabolic syndrome in evening chronotypes." *Scientific Reports* 8, no. 1 (2018): p. 945.

Vernarelli, J.A., D.C. Mitchell, B.J. Rolls, and T.J. Hartman. "Dietary energy density is associated with obesity and other biomarkers of chronic disease in US adults." *European Journal of Nutrition* 54, no. 1 (2015): pp. 59–65.

Versteeg, R.I., A. Schrantee, S.M. Adriaanse, U.A. Unmehopa, J. Booij, L. Reneman, et al. "Timing of caloric intake during weight loss differentially affects striatal dopamine transporter and thalamic serotonin transporter binding." *The FASEB Journal* 31, no. 10 (2017): pp. 4545–4554.

Virtanen, M., A. Singh-Manoux, J.E. Ferrie, D. Gimeno, M.G. Marmot, M. Elovainio, et al. "Long working hours and cognitive function: the Whitehall II Study." *American Journal of Epidemiology* 169, no. 5 (2009): pp. 596–605.

Volkow, N.D., and J.S. Fowler. "Addiction, a disease of compulsion and drive: involvement of the orbitofrontal cortex." *Cerebral Cortex* 10, no. 3 (2000): pp. 318–325.

Volkow, N.D., J.S. Fowler, G.J. Wang, and R.Z. Goldstein. "Role of dopamine, the frontal cortex and memory circuits in drug addiction:

insight from imaging studies." *Neurobiology of Learning and Memory* 78, no. 3 (2002): pp. 610–624.

Volkow, N.D., J.S. Fowler, G.J. Wang, J.M. Swanson, and F. Telang. "Dopamine in drug abuse and addiction: results of imaging studies and treatment implications." *Archives of Neurology* 64, no. 11 (2007): pp. 1575–1579.

Volkow, N.D., G.J. Wang, J.S. Fowler, D. Tomasi, and F. Telang. "Addiction: beyond dopamine reward circuitry." *Proceedings of the National Academy of Sciences of the United States of America* 108, no. 37 (2011): pp. 15037–15042.

Volkow, N.D., R.A. Wise, and R. Baler. "The dopamine motive system: implications for drug and food addiction." *Nature Reviews Neuroscience* 18, no. 12 (2017): pp. 741–752.

Vollaard, N.B.J., and R.S. Metcalfe. "Research into the Health Benefits of Sprint Interval Training Should Focus on Protocols with Fewer and Shorter Sprints." *Sports Medicine* 47, no. 12 (2017): pp. 2443–2451.

Vollaard, N.B.J., R.S. Metcalfe, and S. Williams. "Effect of Number of Sprints in an SIT Session on Change in V O2max: A Meta-analysis." *Medicine & Science in Sports & Exercise* 49, no. 6 (2017): pp. 1147–1156.

von Bartheld, C.S., J. Bahney, and S. Herculano-Houzel. "The search for true numbers of neurons and glial cells in the human brain: A review of 150 years of cell counting." *Journal of Comparative Neurology* 524, no. 18 (2016): pp. 3865–3895.

Wallace, C.W., and S.C. Fordahl. "Obesity and dietary fat influence dopamine neurotransmission: exploring the convergence of metabolic state, physiological stress, and inflammation on dopaminergic control of food intake." *Nutrition Research Reviews* 35, no. 2 (2021): pp. 1–42.

Wang, G.J., N.D. Volkow, and J.S. Fowler. "The role of dopamine in motivation for food in humans: implications for obesity." Expert Opinion on Therapeutic Targets 6, no. 5 (2002): pp. 601–609.

Wang, G.J., N.D. Volkow, J. Logan, N.R. Pappas, C.T. Wong, W. Zhu, et al. Brain dopamine and obesity." *The Lancet* 357, no. 9253 (2001): pp. 354–357.

Wang, M.E., B.K. Singh, M.C. Hsu, C. Huang, P.M. Yen, L.S. Wu, et al. "Increasing Dietary Medium-Chain Fatty Acid Ratio Mitigates High-fat Diet-Induced Non-Alcoholic Steatohepatitis by Regulating Autophagy." *Scientific Reports* 7, no. 1 (2017): p. 13999.

Weinstein, A., A. Livny, and A. Weizman. "New developments in brain research of internet and gaming disorder." *Neuroscience & Biobehavioral Reviews* 75 (2017): pp. 314–330.

"What is Mental Illness?" American Psychiatric Association. https://www.psychiatry.org/patients-families/what-is-mental-illness (accessed April 22, 2024).

White, Ellen G. *The Adventist Home*. Hagerstown, MD: Review and Herald Publishing Association, 1952.

———. *Child Guidance*. Washington, D.C.: Review and Herald Publishing Association, 1954.

———. *Christ's Object Lessons*. Washington, D.C.: Review and Herald Publishing Association, 1900.

———. *Counsels on Diet and Foods*. Washington, D.C.: Review and Herald Publishing Association, 1938.

———. *Counsels on Health*. Mountain View, CA: Pacific Press Publishing Association, 1923.

———. *Daughters of God*. Hagerstown, MD: Review and Herald Publishing Association, 1998.

———. "Degeneracy—Education." *The Health Reformer*, November 1, 1872.

———. *The Desire of Ages*. Mountain View, CA: Pacific Press Publishing Association, 1898.

———. *Education*. Mountain View, CA: Pacific Press Publishing Association, 1903.

———. *The Faith I Live By*. Washington, D.C.: Review and Herald Publishing Association, 1958.

———. *Gospel Workers*. Washington, D. C.: Review and Hearld Publishing Association, 1915.

———. *The Great Controversy*. Mountain View, California: Pacific Press Publishing Association, 1911.

———. *Healthful Living*. Battle Creek, MI: Medical Missionary Board, 1897.

———. *Manuscript Releases*. Vol. 3. Silver Spring, MD: Ellen G. White Estate, 1990.

———. *Manuscript Releases*. Vol. 7. Silver Spring, MD: Ellen G. White Estate, 1990.

———. *Manuscript Releases*. Vol. 12. Silver Spring, MD: Ellen G. White Estate, 1990.

———. *Medical Ministry*. Mountain View, CA: Pacific Press Publishing Association, 1932.

———. *Mind, Character, and Personality*. Vol. 1. Nashville, TN: Southern Publishing Association, 1977.

———. *The Ministry of Healing*. Mountain View, CA: Pacific Press Publishing Association, 1905.

———. *My Life Today*. Washington, D.C.: Review and Hearld Publishing Association, 1952.

———. "The Necessity for Immediate Action." *Sanitarium Announcement*, January 1, 1900.

———. *Patriarchs and Prophets*. Washington, D.C.: Review and Herald Publishing Association, 1890.

———. *Reflecting Christ*. Hagerstown, MD: Review and Herald Publishing Association, 1985.

———. *The Retirement Years*. Hagerstown, MD: Review and Hearld Publishing Association, 1990.

———. *Selected Messages*. Book 2. Washington, D.C.: Review and Herald Publishing Association, 1958.

———. *A Solemn Appeal*. Battle Creek, MI: Seventh-day Adventist Publishing Association, 1870.

———. *Temperance*. Mountain View, CA: Pacific Press Publishing Association, 1949.

———. *Testimonies for the Church*. Vol. 3. Mountain View, CA: Pacific Press Publishing Association, 1875.

———. *Testimonies to Ministers and Gospel Workers*. Mountain View, CA: Pacific Press Publishing Association, 1923.

———. *Thoughts from the Mount of Blessing*. Mountain View, CA: Pacific Press Publishing Association, 1896.

White, P.D., K.A. Goldsmith, A.L. Johnson, L. Potts, R. Walwyn, J.C. DeCesare, et al. "Comparison of adaptive pacing therapy, cognitive behaviour therapy, graded exercise therapy, and specialist medical care for chronic fatigue syndrome (PACE): a randomised trial." *The Lancet* 377, no. 9768 (2011): pp. 823–836.

Wikipedia. 2024. "Chaos Theory." Wikimedia Foundation. Last modified February 16, 2024. https://en.wikipedia.org/wiki/Chaos_theory.

Wikipedia. 2024. "Second Law of Thermodynamics." Wikimedia Foundation. Last modified February 6, 2024. https://en.wikipedia.org/wiki/Second_law_of_thermodynamics.

Wikoff, D., B.T. Welsh, R. Henderson, G.P. Brorby, J. Britt, E. Myers, et al. "Systematic review of the potential adverse effects of caffeine consumption in healthy adults, pregnant women, adolescents, and children." *Food and Chemical Toxicology* 109, pt. 1 (2017): pp. 585–648.

Willett, W.C. "Dietary fats and coronary heart disease." *Journal of Internal Medicine* 272, no. 1 (2012): pp. 13–24.

Wilmore, D.W. "Postoperative protein sparing." *World Journal of Surgery* 23, no. 6 (1999): pp. 545–552.

Wray, N.R., S. Ripke, M. Mattheisen, M. Trzaskowski, E.M. Byrne, A. Abdellaoui, et al. "Genome-wide association analyses identify 44 risk variants and refine the genetic architecture of major depression." *Nature Genetics* 50, no. 5 (2018): pp. 668–681.

Wright, J., J. Kennedy-Stephenson, C. Wang, M. McDowell, and C. Johnson. "Trends in Intake of Energy and Macronutrients—United States, 1971–2000." *Morbidity and Mortality Weekly Report* 53, no. 4 (2004): pp. 80–82.

Wu, W.K., C.C. Chen, P.Y. Liu, S. Panyod, B.Y. Liao, P.C. Chen, et al. "Identification of TMAO-producer phenotype and host-diet-gut dysbiosis by carnitine challenge test in human and germ-free mice." *Gut* 68, no. 8 (2019): pp. 1439–1449.

Yang, Q., Z. Zhang, E.W. Gregg, W.D. Flanders, R. Merritt, and F.B. Hu. "Added sugar intake and cardiovascular diseases mortality among US adults." *JAMA Internal Medicine* 174, no. 4 (2014): pp. 516–524.

Yeung, J.W.K., Z. Zhang, and T.Y. Kim. "Volunteering and health benefits in general adults: cumulative effects and forms." *BMC Public Health* 18, no. 1 (2017): p. 8.

Yin, Z., and D.J. Klionsky. "Intermittent time-restricted feeding promotes longevity through circadian autophagy." *Autophagy* 18, no. 3 (2022): pp. 471–472.

Yockey, H.P. "A calculation of the probability of spontaneous biogenesis by information theory." *Journal of Theoretical Biology* 67, no. 3 (1977): pp. 377–398.

Yockey, H.P. "On the information content of cytochrome c." *Journal of Theoretical Biology* 67, no. 3 (1977): pp. 345–376.

Yu, S., J.W. Yarnell, P.M. Sweetnam, and L. Murray. "What level of physical activity protects against premature cardiovascular death? The Caerphilly study." *Heart* 89, no. 5 (2003): pp. 502–506.

Zada, D., I. Bronshtein, T. Lerer-Goldshtein, Y. Garini, and L. Appelbaum. "Sleep increases chromosome dynamics to enable reduction of accumulating DNA damage in single neurons." *Nature Communications* 10, no. 1 (2019): p. 895.

Zeeni, N., C. Dagher-Hamalian, H. Dimassi, and W.H. Faour. "Cafeteria diet-fed mice is a pertinent model of obesity-induced organ damage: a potential role of inflammation." *Inflammation Research* 64, no. 7 (2015): pp. 501–512.

Zhang, R., P. Manza, and N.D. Volkow. "Prenatal caffeine exposure: association with neurodevelopmental outcomes in 9- to 11-year-old children." *Journal of Child Psychology and Psychiatry* 63, no. 5 (2022): pp. 563–578.

Zhang, W., G. Li, P. Manza, Y. Hu, J. Wang, G. Lv, et al. "Functional Abnormality of the Executive Control Network in Individuals With Obesity During Delay Discounting." *Cerebral Cortex* 32, no. 9 (2022): pp. 2013–2021.

Zhang, Y., F. Li, F.Q. Liu, C. Chu, Y. Wang, D. Wang, et al. "Elevation of Fasting Ghrelin in Healthy Human Subjects Consuming a High-Salt Diet: A Novel Mechanism of Obesity?" *Nutrients* 8, no. 6 (2016): p. 323.

Zheng, B.K., and P.P. Niu. "Higher Coffee Consumption Is Associated With Reduced Cerebral Gray Matter Volume: A Mendelian Randomization Study." *Frontiers in Nutrition* 9 (2022): 850004.

Zheng, X., T. Jiang, H. Wu, D. Zhu, L. Wang, R. Qi, et al. "Hepatic iron stores are increased as assessed by magnetic resonance imaging in a Chinese population with altered glucose homeostasis." *American Journal of Clinical Nutrition* 94, no. 4 (2011): pp. 1012–1019.

Zhong, V.W., L. Van Horn, M.C. Cornelis, J.T. Wilkins, H. Ning, M.R. Carnethon, et al. "Associations of Dietary Cholesterol or Egg Consumption With Incident Cardiovascular Disease and Mortality." *JAMA* 321, no. 11 (2019): pp. 1081–1095.

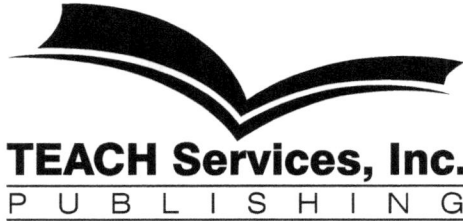

www.ingramcontent.com/pod-product-compliance
Lightning Source LLC
Chambersburg PA
CBHW071052280326
41928CB00050B/2284